Reluctant Human

A Journey Through Two Terminal Diagnoses, Hospice and Healing

Adriana Muñoz Hernández

First published by Ultimate World Publishing 2025

ISBN

Paperback: 978-1-923583-03-0
Ebook: 978-1-923583-04-7

Cover design: Ultimate World Publishing
Layout and typesetting: Ultimate World Publishing
Editor: Rebecca Low
Cover Image Copyrights: Outer Space-Shutterstock.com

ULTIMATE WORLD
— PUBLISHING —

Ultimate World Publishing
Diamond Creek,
Victoria Australia 3089
www.writeabook.com.au

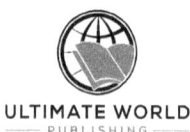

Dedication

I dedicate this book to both Tess Damon and Rev. Tiffany Barsotti.

Tess, you shared our love of art and bravely walked with me down cancer's path. Thank you for teaching me your love and resolve.

Tiffany, I could not have had a better guide. Thank you for your lessons, inspiration, and especially your love.

Contents

Message from the Author

I've included a simple version of an ancient system of codes indicating energetic centers in the body called **chakras***. Throughout this book, I've marked the possible major chakras (energy centers) that have affected my body's balance. When these energetic centers are out of balance, they indicate the body's inability to function properly. They help us guide our health. I think of them like little batteries or electric power sources, like in a house, only they're throughout the body.*

My suggestion to the reader is to note how the energy centers can help us determine where the source of our energy may be blocked as a simple self-check practice. If you've never learned about chakras, this is a truly wonderful way to begin to understand our body.

My goal for this book is to share my experience of surviving against all odds, with the hope that it may help you or someone you know. Everyone's path is complex and different. My life's path was led by my seeking to understand and learn its mysteries. Never leaving a stone unturned eventually took me to Dr. Joe Dispenza. I never met him in person, but I attribute my healing directly to his teachings and meditations. I also learned that there are many ways of healing. My wish is that you'll be inspired to open your mind and heart to the possibility of other ways of healing.

What is a Chakra?

The word "chakra" means spinning disk or wheel of energy that runs down the spine. The health of your chakras directly corresponds with the physical body, the mind, and a person's emotional well-being.

The chakra system originated in India between 1500 and 500 BC in the oldest text called the Vedas.

Anodea Judith, an author and researcher, studied and wrote a book called *The Wheels Of Life*, explaining how the chakra system was passed down through oral tradition. The chakra system and yoga are part of the same system.

Caroline Myss, the well-known author and expert medical intuitive, describes chakras as, "Energy centers within the body that correspond to the distinct stages of human development and spiritual maturation."

Understanding and working with the chakras may be helpful for self awareness.

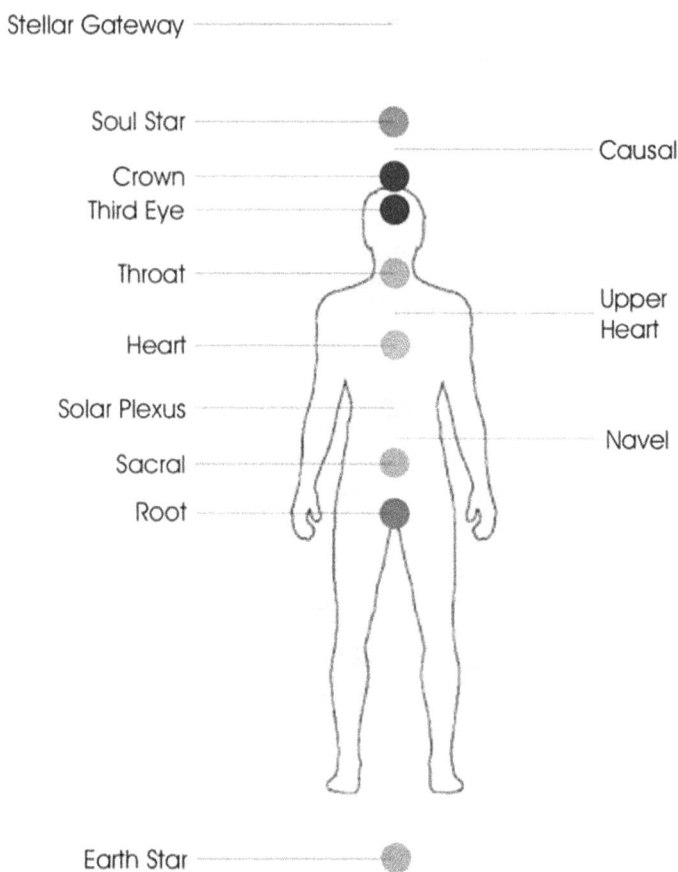

Stellar Gateway

Soul Star

Causal

Crown
Third Eye

Throat

Upper
Heart

Heart

Solar Plexus

Navel

Sacral

Root

Earth Star

Seven Chakra System

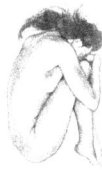

Introduction

I'm what some might call a living miracle. Others may see me as a cat with nine lives. From a very young age, I wanted to understand the mysteries of life. I was a seeker. I believed that anything was possible. I don't know why or where these ideas came from, but I always had a rich inner life.

I've had many journeys, but my most recent and outstanding one began eight years ago in 2017. At the age of 60, I was diagnosed with a very rare, terminal breast cancer—triple-negative metaplastic breast cancer stage 4 (not to be confused with *metastatic).* The prognosis was three years. Eight months later, a new primary cancer located in my brain appeared, glioblastoma multiforme wild type, shortening my life expectancy to 18 months.

Doctors believe that there are three reasons for cancer: genetics, environmental toxins, and constitutional characteristics. While I had no genetic markers for cancer, perhaps an environmental factor may have been an issue. I suspect that accumulated stress and blocked, unaddressed trauma can also result in cancer.

The question is, why am I still alive? I'll attempt to answer this complicated question as best I can.

I'm not a doctor or health professional. I'm an artist and teacher. When I was a young person, I looked for work that was meaningful, as I had a desire to help others. I enjoyed investigating many subjects, but what has intrigued me the most throughout my life is the human condition.

Being a lifelong learner and having an inquisitive mind prepared me to pursue a career in both art and biology. My inherent need for truth came from a deeper and older source that I've only begun to seriously investigate in the last eight years. The source comes from the mystical, unseen truths, where science and mysticism are tethered.

To the amazement of doctors, friends, and family, I'm still alive at the writing of this book, *eight* years later.

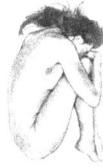

Chapter 1

Mistaken Zygote

*Chakra #1 - Root - Security and stability -
Color: red*

I was born in 1956 in Bogota, Colombia. Childhood memories are usually spotty, ever since I could remember, my body felt tight and uncomfortable. I wanted to break away from it and fly, stretch my wings and soar. It was an uncomfortable and frustrating feeling that would last almost a lifetime. I was a free spirit struggling to embody. Ever since I could remember, there was a missing bond or connection between my parents and I.

Clarissa Pinkola Estes is an American writer and Jungian psychologist. In one of her most famous books, *Women Who Run with the Wolves*, she writes a short story called "Story of the Mistaken Zygote". It explains exactly how I felt growing up.

According to Pinkola Estes, there are women who feel, throughout their lives, that they "dance to a different drummer." She tells a story about a mistaken zygote. The zygote has a "zygote fairy" who carries a fertilized egg in the sky. When it's time, the fairy puts the zygote in a basket to be delivered to the appropriate parents. But, since the zygote is jumping around with the excitement of coming to a family, it falls out of the basket and to the wrong parents.

This was me—I related profoundly to this story.

The wild woman archetype is often found in families that don't understand their daughters. The parents find it difficult to raise them. The daughters are usually seen as headstrong and not allowed to speak to women like them.

Home in Colombia

Chakra #4 - Heart - Love and compassion -
Color: green

I don't know if my mother knew or even suspected she had the wrong "zygote" or not, but the need for forceps to pull me out may have provided a good clue.

Many years later, when I was pregnant with my son, I asked her what my birth was like. She simply said, "The doctor had to use forceps. You didn't want to come out." The indentation left on my jaw is still there to prove it!

I was her first child. My brother came next, then two more boys. Although I was a welcomed baby, her preference for boys was evident. The matriarch made sure to enforce her troops. It became common knowledge to her friends that I was more difficult than the three boys combined.

My parents believed that children were not to be seen or heard. It was a common reminder, especially when there were visitors. Then, it expanded to include, "Children were not to speak to adults unless spoken to."

One day after kindergarten graduation, my parents started moving furniture. This activity was unusual. I had never seen them move the furniture. I noticed that everything was stacked in the center of the apartment's front room. A few minutes later, people entered our small apartment, another unusual sight since we rarely had visitors. Frightened, I asked my mother what was happening. Strangers were entering the small apartment and looking at our things.

"What are they doing?" I asked my mother.

Angrily, she ordered me to be silent.

"But what's happening?" I pleaded!

I knew she was really mad because she did that pinching and twisting thing on my arm as she ordered me to my room.

Even more frightened, I quietly peeked behind the door, crying as I saw people taking away my favorite things, like the painted rainbow colored stool where I sat to read. I would also stand on it so I could reach out of our third-story apartment windows, while the school children passed by on their way to school. I couldn't wait to get the blue and white uniform and knee-high white socks, too!

My mother's sewing machine went next. A very large man folded the table and made it disappear. It was where I made drawings for school. I couldn't bear to look any longer. As I cried myself to sleep, I hoped to wake up and find out it was all a dream. The next morning, when I woke up, it was all real. My parents said we were going to go on an airplane the next day and couldn't take big things with us. So many things that meant home to me were gone. I was shocked and scared. I didn't want to go anywhere.

It wasn't the first time that I had been surprised and scared. In the past, I had awakened in the middle of the night with a nightmare, only to find my parents' unslept bed. I had been left with my grandmother, but the housekeeper stayed with me most of the time. My parents went on trips, thinking it was best not to tell me because I would cry. Thus, I learned at a young age that I couldn't trust them. I felt unsafe, scared, abandoned, and angry.

Although they may not have intended to make me feel abandoned or unloved, this belief was fixed in my brain as such. The lack of communication and mixed messages began around three years old.

The experience of seeing our belongings being taken stayed in my mind for years to come. An unexplained part of me shut down. Perhaps the magic of childhood had ended at that very moment. I became increasingly quiet and vigilant.

My parents said nothing; I said nothing. The horror of seeing my little world taken away without any explanation was hidden. What remained was the beginning of stress, anxiety, and anger building up inside me. From that day on, I lost my sense of home and safety. Becoming unattached to material things prepared me for future loss. After the end of the school year, we left Colombia for the "Land of Opportunity".

What is Trauma?

From the dictionary: Greek word meaning "wound".

Dr. Gabor Maté, a renowned medical doctor and researcher, explains that trauma isn't just an event itself; it's the harm experienced internally due to a challenging circumstance, rather than the circumstance itself.

Unable to understand or use the words to express their emotions, children's brains log traumatic events into their "memory banks" and move on. They don't experience the awareness of the event/trauma that happened to them until later in life. As our brains grow and become more mature, memories may be triggered from infancy. Most of the challenges in life originate in childhood.

As I matured, rather than thinking that I was a victim, as I had thought in the past, I began to view the troubling event as an opportunity to learn from the experience, a sign I was beginning to "awaken".

No longer wanting to live with anger or pain from the past, I chose to learn to see experiences from a different point of view. I had lived attached to the painful emotions of the past for a very long time, continuing to perpetuate the victim narrative.

Finally, learning to heal these feelings by viewing the memory or event without judgment (granted, not easy) or protecting my ego, I started to understand that life is a process of learning. One of the things I needed to do was decode the memories and data in order to understand the lesson. Now I see trauma as an alert mechanism that's signaling our entire body, mind, and spirit to pay attention.

Some scientists say that trauma may originate in the mother's womb. Others cite generational trauma that can continue to be passed down to several generations in a row. They suggest that when a person becomes aware of these embedded family traumas, the patient may be able to resolve/heal an entire family's generational trauma. The healing and releasing of the trauma ensures future members of the family are freed of past generational suffering.

I believe that we've all had our share of trauma that may have originated in childhood. We may even accumulate more as we continue in life. For some, it may take an "awakening" of sorts or professional help to access the subconscious mind. Unresolved trauma blocks emotions that build up over time. Buried deep into our psyche, stress, anxiety, or fear eventually produces toxic chemicals that get stored in our bodies. Eventually, if unresolved, these depleting emotions get blocked and manifest in illness in both children and adults.

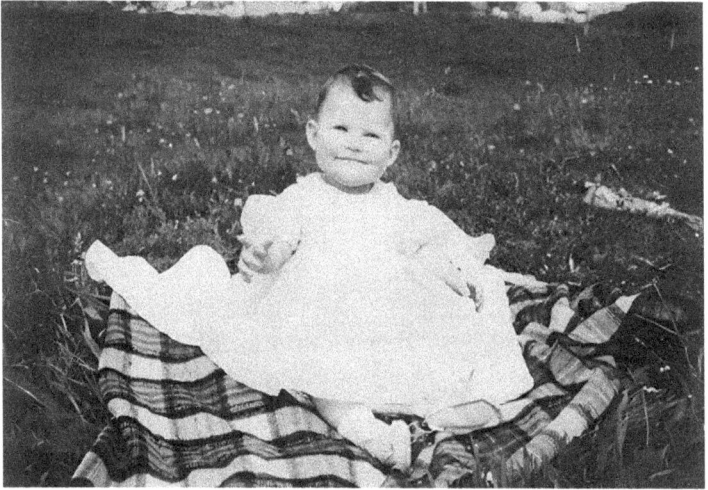

Author at one year old

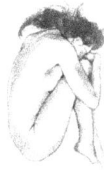

Chapter 2

American Dream

Chakra #1 - Security and stability - Color: red
Chakra #2 - Creativity and emotions - Color: orange

My memory of our trip to the United States, particularly the seven-hour flight from Bogota, Colombia, to LAX, is spotty. I can only surmise that it must have been a midnight flight, and I slept the entire time, or that it was another traumatic event my brain refuses to remember.

My father's Dutch boss at KLM Airlines in Colombia, who had also emigrated to the US, sponsored us. Upon arriving, my father held tight to the four resident visas in his hand. We walked together to a fancy phone booth. My father came out of the booth shocked. He had received terrible news. His superior had just been arrested for embezzling from the company. Appalled and afraid, he took us to our new home.

Our new apartment in the U.S. was larger than our Colombian apartment. But I was surprised to see a double mattress in the middle of what looked like the living room floor. That's where we all slept together the first night. We weren't rich in Colombia, but we weren't poor either. To my six-year-old self, we looked very poor now. There was no furniture, no colorful wooden stool to sit on.

My father was embarrassed and afraid. He didn't dare to show up at his new office for fear of being associated with the man who had sponsored him. He had to look for another job immediately. He took the first job he found and started work at a radiator company in South Central, Los Angeles. The factory was on strike, but he broke the line in desperation and remained employed until 65 without a pension.

The first six months in the U.S. passed quickly. My brother and I were allowed to play with our next-door neighbors' children, a welcome new experience.

My parents and many other immigrants in the 1960s were seeking the American Dream—social progress, increased power of acquisition, better opportunities for work, security, better schools, and less corruption. They had ambition for a promising future. For my brother and I, it was another story.

Entering first grade in the U.S. was bittersweet. I had waited so long for this moment to arrive, but the first friend I made was in kindergarten, and I looked forward to being in the same class with her again. When I realized I would never see her again, the joy, like a big red balloon, burst in my heart. Thankfully, I remembered that my mother had told me that morning that we were going to have another baby in the house. Maybe I would get a baby sister to play with, I hoped!

My mother didn't speak English. It took a long time for her to lose the shame of speaking with a thick accent. Luckily, I inherited my father's ability for languages, so I was already speaking English after six months. Therefore, I was delegated to be her translator when my father wasn't home. It felt good to do something she approved of.

Although my mother had worked in a bank when she was single, she didn't expect to work as a married woman. In Colombia, even a middle-class family could afford someone to help with house chores. My mother had been raised in a large family with three or more housemaids who helped raise her 11 siblings as well as cook and clean. Now she was faced with having to do it all herself with a third child, a rude awakening. We became latch-key kids, and I was expected to come home from school to feed my brothers and make rice for that evening's dinner.

My mother may not have been the perfect mother, a great housekeeper, a fantastic cook, or highly educated, but she was smart, practical, resolute, intuitive, resourceful, and emotionally strong.

My father was a gentleman—traditional, polished, somewhat intellectual, passive, religiously conservative, and proper, but mostly fearful. He valued knowledge, ethics, and morals. His intentions were good, as were my mother's, but they were mostly inflexible and very strict.

I cannot begin to imagine how my parents must have negotiated their own fears and misgivings when coming to the United States in 1962. They had no support system, no extended family.

Since my father was a strict Roman Catholic, a Catholic education was imperative. My skin was a very light shade, and I thought I looked like the other children. One day in third grade, I was going out to recess, and the girls were talking about a party one of them was having. The birthday girl began giving out the invitations. I was excited with the anticipation of attending my first birthday party in the US. As the girls gathered around each other, I joined them. The birthday girl came closer. I was surely next! But she missed me; she didn't give me an invitation!

"Excuse me," I said politely, "You missed me!"

"Yes," she continued proudly, "My mother said you can't go to my party."

I sheepishly asked her why.

"Because my mother says you're Mexican."

I "understood" because my mother didn't let me talk to Mexicans either.

"I'm not Mexican! I'm Colombian!" I protested.

"It doesn't matter! My mother says you have a Mexican name, so you're still Mexican," she snapped. I was crushed.

That's when I realized that I wasn't like the others. I didn't belong. Although we had been taught that Jesus had said, "Love others as yourself," clearly this was one of those rules that was only meant for "those of your own kind." We were told, I thought, that "everyone was equal." Another truth debunked. Another point for the "reluctant human".

Becoming aware that I was different set up a pattern of thought that I was unworthy. This is an example of how my brain put this information together.

- *The information my brain received first was that I was **different**.*
- *Being **different** = rejected, I don't belong.*
- *Since I was **rejected**, I was considered **unacceptable**.*
- ***Different = rejection***
- ***Different = unaccepted***

- *The **feeling** of being **rejected** or being **unaccepted**, led to the **validation** of the **thought** that I was **unworthy**.*
- *Therefore, the **pattern** of **feeling rejected** and **thinking** I was **unworthy** was initiated.*

A seemingly endless loop is created. Remember, our brains dislike change. That's why it's difficult to remove that block. If the pattern is repeated often enough, you begin to believe it. Then it becomes part of your personality. This is why meditation or hypnosis is a good way to remove blocks.

Adding these new thoughts validated my belief of unworthiness that I felt from my parents. I was not only not good enough for my family but also not good enough for my schoolmates.

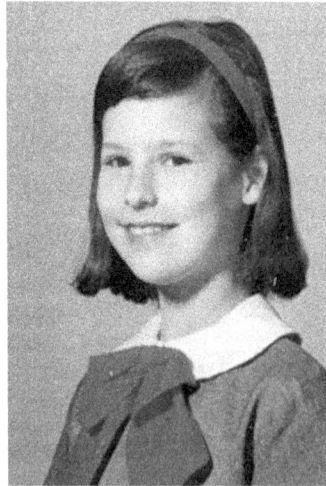

Author in third grade

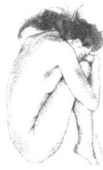

Chapter 3

I Feel You

Chakra #2 - Creativity and emotions - Color: orange
Chakra #3 - Personal power and confidence -
Color: yellow

I was a sensitive child who felt things intensely. The range of feelings I had as a child was more varied and nuanced than all the colors in the rainbow. Solid pigments of infinite colors, like in a box of 100 Crayons with their many hues and values, are closer to the complex ideas and emotions I felt. The expression of my emotions that filled my inner world became a source of punishment and humiliation as my parents and brothers found it either annoying or entertaining.

As I became older and was exposed to more of the world and its humans, I felt confused and disappointed to witness the reality of good and evil. It's one of the mysteries I've grappled with all my life. Overwhelmed with the world's injustice, like poverty, killing, wars, etc., worry and helplessness constantly occupied my mind. I didn't know how to help. The only thing I could do was continue learning in school and books, seeking to understand what I came here for. Feeling everything so deeply at such a young age, as if the world's problems were my own, I felt helpless and tired. But I didn't know why. Maybe there was something wrong with me.

It would be many years later that I would find out I was an empath. I didn't know the word "empath" when I was nine, but in my journey to better health, I've learned a few things.

People who are "empaths" are identified by the following characteristics:

- *Feeling a shift in mood when someone enters a room or space*
- *Needing to spend weeks alone in order to recharge*
- *When you're in the presence of "energy vampires" (someone you find exhausting or takes your energy), you feel drained of energy, exhausted*

It's one thing to have empathy for people or be sensitive to other people's feelings. It's another thing to feel extremely exhausted mentally, physically, or emotionally. We're beings made of energy.

Emotional energy is manifested or felt as a vibration. When you're an empath, you're tuned in (like a radio) and more sensitive to the energy around you. Your own energy is sensitive and is therefore affected by it.

There are different levels of energy:

Level 1: Knower

A **knower** senses what people around them are feeling. They may not necessarily absorb the emotions of others, but they can easily become overwhelmed in large groups of people. This type of empath is **mentally depleting**.

Level 2: Feeler

A **feeler** tunes into the emotions that other people are experiencing. They feel someone else's emotion and therefore confuse it as their own. The **feeler** finds themselves with a feeling they don't recognize, wondering where that emotion came from when in fact, it was someone else's. They feel depleted or tired around certain people, mistaking it as their tiredness or sadness. This type of energy empath is **emotionally depleting**.

Level 3: Embodied

An **embodied** empath can actually feel the physical pain of others. They may be around someone with an injury and suddenly have the pain associated with it. This type of empath is **physically depleting**.

Empaths are especially vulnerable to experiencing energetic blocks that prevent them from showing up in the world because of how sensitive they are. These energetic blocks can show up as mental illness, physical ailments, financial problems, relationship issues, feeling "stuck", lack of purpose, lack of confidence, anxiety, depression, or just a general feeling of unhappiness.

If you identify with some of these traits, it's important to find ways to protect yourself. Just like we protect ourselves from things we cannot see, like electricity, X-rays, 5G, electromagnetic, and other energy, there are tools to protect ourselves.

Our bodies are made of energy. We literally have an energetic field inside of us and around us. Light also has an energy field.

You can create a protective field using visualization to shield the energy around you.

You can choose different colors of light while you visualize the shield descending from above. The colors you choose can saturate your shield, creating a vibrant and impenetrable barrier.

You can also visualize a protective shield by closing your eyes and imagining your own energy developing in a protective shield. Visualize this shield as a powerful barrier that filters out negative energies while allowing positive energies to flow through. Experiment with different shapes to see what resonates with you, whether it's a bubble, pyramid, spiral, sphere, etc.

Intention and prayer are other forms of protection. They're simple but powerful, allowing you to establish a positive and protective energy around you. Some people choose to pray to God, goddesses, a higher power, the universe, etc. There's no right or wrong way to do this.

Looking to understand the existence of good and evil, I found possible explanations from philosophical, religious, and metaphysical perspectives.

Ancient Egyptian mythology gives us the first example of murder with the killing of the god Osiris by his brother Set, revealing the struggle between good and evil.

Christian religious teachings, in general, regard good and evil as a result of Adam and Eve partaking in the forbidden fruit. Cain's murder of his brother Abel was another incident that depicted God's wrath (parallels some of the Egyptian myths and several other religions).

*In metaphysics, we're presented with the concept that we live in a world of duality, up and down, light and dark, good and evil—evil being the absence or presence of light. Having free will, we're free to decide what spectrum of evil/darkness we choose to be on. God doesn't **create** evil. Our reality needs the assurance of comparisons in order to learn.*

We're free to choose to follow the path of light or the path of darkness. There's no good or evil as such; it's just a descriptor in the existence of the duality. The Universe, God, gods, Allah, goddess—whatever you want to call it, is always light. God is light. Darkness is ignorance, lack of light, or lack of knowing. Evil isn't created by a God or other deity. In metaphysics, the fundamentaul question of reality, the nature of consciousness, and God are frequently explored.

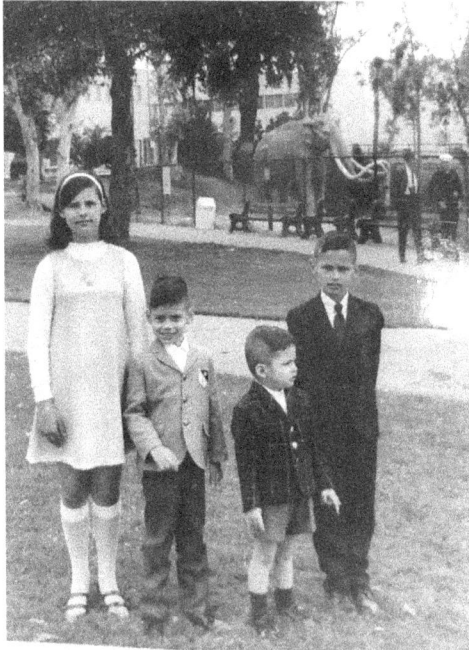

Authors' brothers

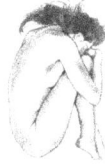

Chapter 4

Assimilation vs. Acculturation

Chakra #1 - Root-grounding, stability,
survival - Color: red
Chakra #2 - Sacral-creativity, sexual and
emotional balance - Color: orange
Chakra #3 - Solar Plexus - personal power,
confidence, self-esteem - Color: yellow

Being an immigrant presented a complicated problem that added to my being a six-year-old reluctant human. When we arrived in the United States in 1962, there weren't as many immigrants coming from Mexico or South America as there are now. We were still the minority. The system for legal immigrants to adapt to the new culture was assimilation. This system causes immigrants to abandon their own culture in order to become part of the greater group. Immigrants were encouraged to follow the American way of living by the "white" American society. Attempting to become part of the American system, immigrants often began to reject their own culture, which not only affects the interaction of people of different races but also leads to a dilemma within one's race. The process forces immigrants to lose their identity.

Assimilation rates have increased over time. A larger generation gap among immigrants has also increased. The younger generation seems enthusiastic to embrace American culture in order to be accepted. In contrast, the older immigrants are left to worry about preserving their traditions.

In order to cope with the nostalgia, some immigrant families choose rather to **acculturate.** Reluctant to lose their original heritage, these immigrants accept the new host country's culture while still retaining the traditions of their origins.

Since I was seen as different, I was hesitant to participate in class or even talk to the other children. Fearful that they would judge me because of my background, I was mostly quiet throughout the early years of grade school. In order to ease my feeling of being an outsider, I chose to assimilate into the American lifestyle. I built a relationship with other students whose parents were from other countries.

I believe that in my parents' case, they didn't foresee the difficulty they would be presented with when raising their children and maintaining their Hispanic identity. Perhaps that's the origin of the many mixed messages my brothers and I received while growing up. They wanted to raise us under the rules and traditions of Colombian culture, while also assimilating to American culture. Unfortunately, the difficulty of integrating our identities was too overwhelming. In fact, it may have been difficult for them personally as well; therefore, it makes sense that there were so many mixed messages. Unfortunately, their own desire to assimilate resulted in the loss of their own traditions and cultural heritage. I was in two conflicting realities.

Identity

Leaving Colombia when I was a child was a traumatic experience. Leaving my grandmothers, cousins, and aunts was impossible for me to understand. Communication with my extended family was inconsistent. The first time I returned to Colombia was when I was 15 years old. Reconnecting with my cousins was identity-affirming. I felt I was finally back home.

When I visited again at 17, I wanted to stay, but I had to start college right after I turned 18 that summer in Colombia. Then, I went back one last time for almost a year, hoping to stay permanently. To my dismay, I realized that it wouldn't be possible. It wouldn't be acceptable for me to live alone or with a roommate while having so many family members that I could live with. "Good girls" simply didn't live alone or with roommates. There was no other option but to return to the US.

These few visits to my country of birth gave me a little more clarity about myself. Meeting so many different relatives and even seeing people in the streets who looked like me gave me a sense of connection that I had missed.

I could tell that there was something in my family that held something for me to learn.

As I got older, the different cultural and social expectations at home, in addition to those of the American culture that I was growing up in, fueled my anger and disconnect. My parents' rules were based on the social norms of a society still living in the past, perpetuating religious customs, politics, and the results of the instability of an almost 50-year civil war. Well aware of the expectations my parents had for their only female child, I tried to please them, but I had come into this world rebellious and would never be the "right" zygote.

The emerging changes in morality, antiwar rhetoric, and the hippie movement in the U.S. were diametrically opposed to the reality my parents came from. These changes had not yet caught on in our home country.

In the 1960s and 70s in the U.S., young women began to question their roles in society. In the past, only two aspects of femininity were acceptable. The first was becoming a mother whose primary purpose in life was to care for everyone and everything. The second was the maiden, who knew nothing and was always sweet, cute, and innocent.

I was a teenager in the 70s when the women's movement was still going strong. Young women like me were being exposed to art, cinema, and literature that challenged the meaning of women's roles. Young men and women began to move away from religious teachings and challenge the social norms of the past. Amidst this social, moral, and political revolution, many began to find their own values. Women began to look outside the roles delegated to them. They began to venture outside of the old rules.

I didn't completely agree with all of the ideas that were being expressed by the women's movement, but I identified with the desire to be free of traditional women's roles.

Surprised to see that paternalism was being played out even in American politics, I rejected the sexist, backward, and perpetuating idea that women were "not good enough". (A concept that had been drilled into me all my life.)

Trying to understand what was "wrong" with me and my rebellious tendencies, made me want to learn more about why people did not question most things. The more I grew up, the more reluctant I became to follow social norms, even the old American norms. My parents' customs concerning morality and social expectations remained the same in their minds, eons away from the fast-changing world of the United States. As my parents were navigating through the difficult task of raising a family with norms they didn't understand nor agree with, I cannot help but imagine how difficult that must have seemed, an impossible task.

Maturity, self-help books, tapes, therapy, having my own child helped me to forgive myself for the rage and impatience I felt. Compassion and empathy helped me understand my parents' faults; their own parents' parenting abilities were dubious. Our parents had followed what they had learned from their own parents.

Would I just succumb to following what my peers are doing? Should I follow the norms of this assimilated culture or of the culture I came from? The answer was neither. Finding my own version of truth was the only answer for me. The act of questioning and investigating has led me to several different paths.

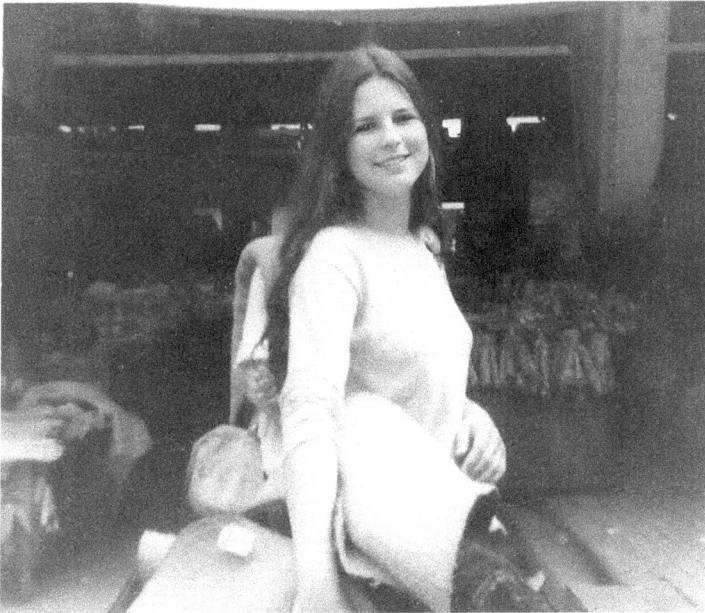

Author age 15 in Colombia

Yoga Practice

Yoga is an ancient practice that originated in Northern India in approximately 1500 BCE. It focuses on uniting the physical self and the spiritual world. In the 19th and 20th centuries, Indian gurus were introduced to the Western world. Modern yoga has evolved into many different styles, while maintaining its ancient roots. It consists of a group of physical, mental, and spiritual practices or disciplines, including postures that increase strength and flexibility.

I was fortunate to have been introduced to yoga in my high school years. Taken aback by the immense sensation of relaxation and calm I felt after class, my love of yoga grew. Although I've always enjoyed dancing and sports, I hadn't developed a conscious relationship with my body yet.

As I've gotten older, and during most of my recoveries, it has been a great source of exercise. The meditation aspect of yoga was the precursor to developing a meditation practice. Through the practice of yoga, I learned the importance of proper breathing, an essential part of all healing.

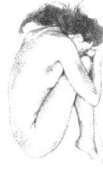

Chapter 5

Love

*Chakra # 5 - Heart-love,
compassion,
and emotional healing -
Color: green*

My first experience of romantic love was when I was in high school. My brothers were older, and I didn't have to run home to cook the obligatory rice anymore. The Los Angeles County Art Museum became my home away from home. It was a place where I

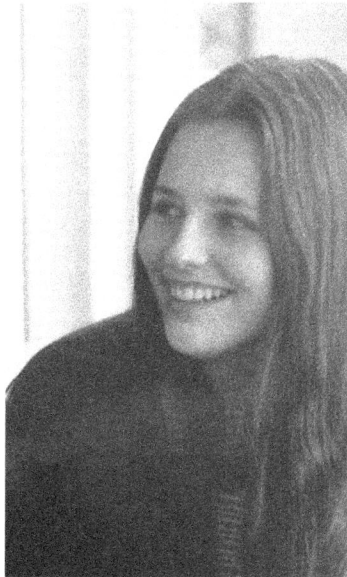

Author at 16 years old

could avoid the noise, my younger brothers' tattling, the TV, and extra chores. It was on the way home on the bus, so I could stop for an hour and then get back on the bus to my house.

I felt happy and serene, eager to see the Caravaggios, Titians, and Rembrandts once again. It became my secret happy place. My father had been the one to introduce us to the museum when we were newly arrived, when I was six. He would take us there periodically throughout the years, but I was now old enough to go by myself. If I had a little extra money, I would go to the museum coffee shop and get some coffee or a snack.

On one of those occasions, I met a 23-year-old man with long, blond hair down to his mid-back, almost as long as mine. His light blue eyes twinkled in the sunlight. He was an aspiring hippy poet, looking for his north star. When he realized I was only 16, it was too late; we were in love. I didn't have the intention of marrying, and much less at a young age. My priority remained to study.

We stayed together for three happy years, then it was time for me to go to university. He was dismayed at my decision to end our relationship and initially hurt, but we were able to maintain our friendship to this day. Fortunate isn't enough to express the gratitude I have for being in one of the most loving, kind, and conscious relationships I've ever had.

A few years into university, I met and fell in love with a 30-year-old man who was divorced and fighting for custody of his six-year-old son. He was very charming but emotionally immature. I was a rescuer, becoming attracted to the first man who showed me love. Based on my initial experience, I assumed other men would have the maturity of my first boyfriend, but I was wrong. I fell in love with falling in love. Confusing love with rescuing someone who needed mothering made me feel worthy. But the opposite occurred; the more I felt needed, the more attracted I was to "help" him. Being loyal to a fault, I stayed in this toxic relationship with the aim of changing him.

During those first three years of university, I was an emotional wreck to the degree that I had to take a year off from school and take refuge in Colombia. After I ended the relationship, I vowed not to get involved until I finished my degree.

When I was 23, a handsome, talented young man and fellow art student joined our studio art class. Let's call him D. We became good friends, and throughout the following two years, we grew close.

Having taken six years to complete two undergraduate programs, one in fine art and the other in biology, I needed a break. D and I started seeing each other more, but there were no discussions of commitment yet. His plan was to take a study abroad program to study Chinese art in Taipei, R.O.C. My plan was to go to Europe and finally visit the Great Masters in person.

Unexpectedly, D invited me to visit him in Taiwan instead. The probability of my visiting Asia or China was slim, much less Taiwan. The opportunity to have this experience wasn't something that I had foreseen, nor did I imagine I would have this opportunity again. I packed my bags and off I went. Both D and I were happy to see each other. I enjoyed learning about a culture so different from ours.

One day, while in Taiwan, I stood waiting at a long traffic light. I was approached by an elegant elderly gentleman. While he briefly talked to me in his thick accent, he was impressed with my non-specific English pronunciation. As the traffic light finally turned, he continued speaking to me. By the time we reached the other side of the street, he had offered me a job teaching English at his private school. Welcoming this once-in-a-lifetime experience wasn't to be missed. The intended two-week visit turned into almost a year.

A year later, D finished his Chinese Art studies program and graduated. He originally planned to try his luck in the Hong Kong art market, but now he found himself undecided. Although I wanted us to return together, I encouraged him to follow his dream.

My dream was to live in the San Francisco Bay area. I was 23 years old, and it was 1979. The Bay Area was not yet the Silicon Valley it has become. The hippie generation had matured, and now it had evolved into the New Age era. Berkeley was a beautiful college town that held a special place in my heart. I met many like-minded people. They seemed open, progressive, introspective, and most of all, fellow seekers.

Defining

I was finally free from my parents and excited to live life on my terms. A few months quickly passed, and to my surprise, D called me from the San Francisco Airport. He was on his way to Berkeley to join me! We happily lived together for two years without marrying, uninterested in following social norms.

Both our parents enjoyed visiting us, but the trouble it took to keep them believing that we didn't live together proved to be too complicated. Every time they wanted to visit, we had to set up an entire production to keep them from finding out the truth. We weren't brave enough to confront them. Unable to be truthful about living together, we decided to get married. We loved each other anyway, so we thought we might as well avoid the stress and hassle. We had a lovely wedding, but in the deep recesses of our unconscious, we knew something else was being played out.

You see, we both knew that there would come a day when we would have to face the possibility of parting ways. Both of us had unresolved issues about our sexuality. We were living during a time and place when the women's movement and changing morality questioned the social norms. Many young people began to explore their sexuality in response to a need for change. Many men and women who had previously been "closeted", hiding their personal lives, now came "out", emboldened by brave leaders. The younger people allowed themselves to live and act openly, while still others began to explore.

Intuitively, I knew that my husband's path would eventually lead to embracing his homosexuality. I was just grateful for whatever time we had together. I had also explored my sexuality, but didn't identify as a lesbian. I was attracted to the person, not the gender. I know, hard for some to understand. During the six years my husband D and I were together, we remained loyal to each other. Mostly, we ignored our other inclinations.

Re-defining

Eventually I built up the courage to confront my fear of rejection as an artist. The many years of unworthiness and fear of rejection or success that I had been building since childhood were deeply rooted. I took classes and workshops to build my self-esteem.

Finally building up courage, I launched myself as a freelance editorial photographer and started exhibiting in galleries, competitions, and art shows. I was doing well and starting to gain a little notoriety, but freelance work was unsteady, which in my mind translated into insecurity and lack of self-worth.

Remembering that the idea of monetizing my artwork had been a conflict for me in the past, my negative thinking turned into self-sabotage. Now all I wanted to do was to run.

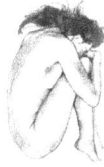

Chapter 6

Taken

Chakras - All seven colors: rainbow

A wave of discontent and insecurity washed over me, and I felt lonely. I missed a sense of connection with my Hispanic identity. When I mentioned this feeling to a long-time friend one day, she acted upon the call.

A few days later, my friend told me that she had just met a Hispanic woman who expressed the exact same feeling. She suggested that maybe we could meet with her new acquaintance. Something about the intensity with which my friend was describing this person felt strange, and I declined.

A few months later, I was looking for a part-time job in a photography studio. Responding to a lead, I met a young Hispanic woman working there. I applied and got the job.

One day, the girl at the photo shop was telling me about her roommate, a woman who reminded her of me. She wanted me to meet her. Surprised once again, I felt a strong negative response that I could not explain. What was happening? I didn't want to meet this woman either! I didn't know why, in addition to rejection, I also detected fear. Never before had I experienced trepidation or anxiety when meeting someone.

Lo and behold, the roommate turned out to be the very same woman I had almost been introduced to by my long-time friend! The serendipity of this event made me extremely uneasy.

A week later, the mystery woman appeared at the photo studio. Her intention was to surprise me by coming in unannounced. I cannot explain the intensity of my antipathy at the moment of seeing her. I had never felt this feeling toward anyone: heart pounding, a need to deny the moment, and full of fear. Dizzy and unsteady, I grabbed the counter for strength.

In the midst of being introduced to this strange woman, my inner voice was screaming NO! I ignored my intuition in favor of engaging and exploring this curious five-legged cat. Clearly, this was an intense, life-changing experience. I didn't understand many of the things that she was talking about, but they were definitely mysterious. I found myself under her spell.

While I questioned myself during this strange moment, I heard myself inviting her to my home to meet my husband. I couldn't believe the words coming out of my mouth.

I was visibly shaking as I spoke. As a Hispanic, I was taught to be polite and extend friendship when introduced by others. But the fact was, I had an absolute 100% repulsion and panic when I met this 45-plus-year-old woman, whom I will refer to as B. She was a lesbian, the embodiment of all my learned and unknown prejudices. She looked and acted like a man—heavy, short, unattractive, masculine, and Mexican. Wearing a black leather bike jacket, black leather motorcycle boots, with straight, short black hair, very white skin, and piercing black eyes.

I didn't understand why I had asked her to come to my home. It was as if I were being led by an invisible force towards her. My world was turned upside down. The basic structure of my life began to crumble.

While I had suspected that my husband, D, would be the first one to end our relationship, it was I who was seduced into exploring a new path. Approximately six months later, my husband and I amicably divorced. He was now happily free to live his authentic life and flourish.

I sold my belongings and headed to Mexico with B. My family wanted nothing to do with me after meeting her; neither did many of my friends. Some of my friends were afraid for me. I was also afraid for myself, but inexplicably, I felt compelled to follow her. Simultaneously, I was challenged by my ego, secretly wanting to unmask her and prove that she was an impostor. Thus began my experience of the Dark Night of the Soul.

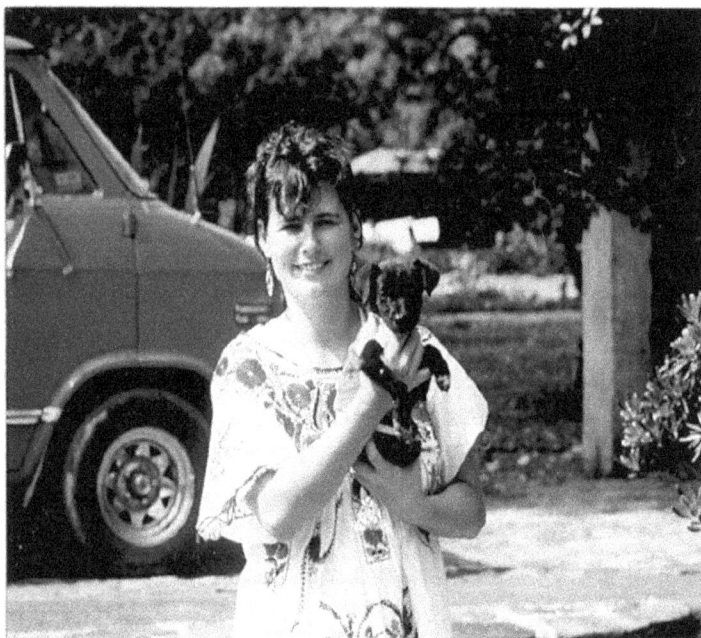

Author at age 30

What is the Dark Night of the Soul?

The Dark Night of the Soul is a spiritual awakening. It's the beginning of a process of liberation from our conditioning by society and family. During this process, we discover the truth about who we really are rather than who others dictate us to be. It's a powerful human experience leading towards the understanding of our true essence. It's painful and challenging because it requires the "cutting of cords" (unseen actual energy) and attachments. In addition, it requires facing and accepting loss. The experience of the Dark Night of the Soul may last from six months to several years. Not everyone experiences a Dark Night of the Soul.

I embarked on a long and dark journey facing an energy that engulfed me in a moment of weakness. I had met my shadow, my mirror, the dark side of me that I had not yet seen.

In my late teens and early 20s, I had no intention of getting married. I didn't want children or to ever be financially dependent on a man. Yet at the age of 30, I had entrusted my power to someone, believing that a fellow woman would never wrong another woman.

Swept Off My Feet

When I first met B, part of me understood that I was involved in a power play that was being enacted as if I were in another reality where I had agreed to play the game. I recognized her as a teacher, a guru, of sorts. Seduced by her "magic", I allowed myself to form a sexual relationship with her. She was gallant in her masculine role of protector. She was the "Knight in Shining Armor", who swept me off my feet and protected me like no man ever had.

Those who saw through her stayed away. I know it sounds unreal, but in fact, she did have the ability to wind her charismatic web of powers around any unsuspecting weak individual.

Don't get me wrong, I don't see myself as a victim. The combination of my hunger for truth, endless curiosity, naiveté, lack of knowledge, and arrogance contributed to the end result of my experience. It was how I unconsciously chose to learn the lesson I needed to learn.

Proclaiming herself as a "Master of Metaphysics" and as an "Ascended Master", she impressed many and was feared by others. What perhaps could have been a six-month exploration into the dark forest of my mind turned into a five-year journey under her training.

Spiritual Boot Camp

Once established in Mexico, B declared that since I had agreed to live with her, it was time to begin what she called "spiritual boot camp". I assumed she was kidding.

B's training included her version of metaphysics, mysticism, and consciousness. It was evident that she indeed had extrasensory gifts. I witnessed her ability to manipulate and disarm several police men, a dangerous rapist, and a home intruder. Even the Mexican "federales" (federal police) softened and submitted to her command. I saw how visibly altered the energy around her environment changed others around her.

At first, we lived in a very small village approximately an hour from Mexico City. According to B, it was considered the "Tibet of Mexico", sister city of Sedona, Arizona. It was truly a mysterious and magical place. I accepted the false fears she subtly fed me until I realized, albeit slowly, that I had surrendered all of my power to someone else's manipulation. The confidence I had acquired in my younger years had disappeared. I now felt constant danger from men, wild dogs, all strangers, and any authority other than her.

One year later, we moved to a large, picturesque town with art schools, a community of artists, and retired expats. Unlike the previous town we had just left, there were many opportunities to meet people and take classes and workshops.

B manipulated me with double-speak and mind games. Every evening, we would go over different levels of reality, and she would repeatedly drill me to change the way I thought. I was compliant because I was committed to becoming a better and happier person. Eventually, I began to suspect her approach once we were living together. I felt that I was losing myself as our entanglement grew. In her presence, things I had known all my life suddenly didn't make sense. I was in a state of confusion.

As my ability to discern awakened, my observation skills increased. To my dismay, I began to see signs of B's wobbly ethics. Although she professed awareness, she was unable to identify the incongruencies of her behavior. Finally, the truth became clear to me. A true spiritual guide wouldn't instill fear or take advantage of someone's vulnerability. Sad for both of us, B was in fact an impostor. Acknowledging this fact provided me the strength to leave my "captor" and the cage I had put myself in.

The tactics of control B practiced are often used in cults, religious groups, wars, and kidnappings. Although she may not have been officially any of those things, she definitely practiced psychological manipulation.

I hadn't been aware of the existence of the dark night of the soul. Confronting that darkness is confusing and frightening, but I believe that becoming aware of its existence and having to face my truth liberated me.

From the depths of the shadows, there's nowhere else to go but back up to the light. The trick is not to get stuck, fall into despair, or give up trying to get back to the light.

It's easy to judge the woman whom I could blame as having "broken" and "kidnapped" my spirit with the promise of enlightenment. I didn't heed the warnings because my ego had something to prove. I learned many invaluable lessons, one of which was learning to be humble. I learned the importance of self-love, something that I hadn't known how to achieve, nor what it really meant. Such simple words, and yet so difficult for me to integrate.

Blaming myself or others is useless. Owning up to my own arrogance, responsibility, and prejudice led me to empower myself. I'm aware that the choices I made may have been dangerous. Nevertheless, it was what my spirit had asked of me. I might as well use what I learned in order to continue my life's journey.

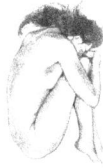

Chapter 7

Who Am I, Really?

Chakra #1 - Root-grounding, stability - Color: red
Chakra #2 - Sacral-creativity and emotion -
Color: orange
Chakra #3 - Solar Plexus - personal power,
confidence - Color: yellow

The popular author and professor, Joseph Campbell, wrote a book called *The Hero's Journey*, which became a series on PBS several years ago. He explains the role of archetypes beautifully. But it was the work of the famous psychologist, Carl Jung, who developed the practice of using archetypes for understanding human behavior.

Archetypes are a source of information that can help guide the understanding of the origin of our behaviors and thoughts. Discovering that we have been programmed to behave, think, expect, and believe was remarkable and frankly shocking!

Surprisingly, I found that the origin of some of my long-held beliefs about love, social roles, and behaviors was clearly represented in Jung's list, which made me realize how predictable we human beings can be. It turns out that much of our behavior has been learned through the embedded patterns established in the past. As ideas and customs developed throughout generations, they established themselves in cultural norms. Not exactly surprising, but definitely not something that I had been aware of.

Taken aback to see how my "archetypes" clearly described my family myths and beliefs explained so much! Becoming aware of them prepared me to consciously begin to change unwanted behaviors.

The process of identifying our archetypes can be difficult at first. You have to be willing to be honest with yourself and refrain from judgment. All of the archetypes have a positive and negative aspect to them. The possibility that you may find aspects of yourself that you may not like or want to accept is to be expected. Going through the process of checking ourselves reveals interesting family, cultural, social, or thought patterns that were learned. It can reveal an aspect of ourselves that we have mistaken for a trait when, in fact, it's an embedded learned behavior.

Behaviors are how a person acts, while personality is a person's very nature or character. In short, we learn behaviors, but we are born with personality.

If we get stuck on an unwanted behavior, then we can access this tool to check and see if it's coming from a hidden pattern or something else. The study of archetypes revealed why I was conflicted with thoughts and intuitions. Knowing that our faults may have come from subconscious patterns helped me to release some of my negative self-talk by realizing that the origin of my belief was based on a repeating family pattern.

Our brains follow patterns that are embedded in our subconscious, and since our brains don't like change, it takes a lot of energy to change. Just like a computer, it will refuse to do what you want it to do unless it has the proper "program" or "software". It may even shut down. It's not uncommon to live an entire life unaware of the prison of programmed thoughts.

Eager to work on letting go of negative patterns, the urgency to resolve them felt like the urge to eliminate parasites from my body. Embracing the discomfort of change while practicing to change has empowered me. With the goal of finding my authentic self, I steadily moved forward.

With some unease, I sometimes think, could there be a deeper force that has been entrusted to maintain and control our behavior?

When I realized that I had attached myself to a "storybook-like" romantic love archetype, like Cinderella, waiting for my elusive "knight in shining armor" to arrive, I immediately saw at least one of the patterns I had been playing out with B. No wonder I had felt so "swept off my feet"! B had been playing the role of the "knight" and I was the "unloved maiden"!

I couldn't help but feel a little angry and maybe even scammed by the beliefs I had been attached to. I was completely unaware of the hidden subconscious roles I was acting out. "Who the hell had put this crap into my head?" I asked myself. "Why did I buy into what I knew better to avoid?"

This reminds me of when I was studying art in university. We were introduced to advertising design classes. Artists have always used psychological tools to alter or change reality. The goal in advertising was to make something super attractive or desirable in order to stand out. As consumerism increased, so did the unethical nature of advertisements. The subliminal messages from these advertisements have gotten stronger and more pervasive. In our current world, we're all bombarded with images and memes that are far from real, creating a confusing world.

I believe advances in technology are fabulous, but I fear the focus on using it is quickly destroying the fabric of our culture. Can we learn to carefully discern the truth and actually rely more on our inner knowledge or intuition?

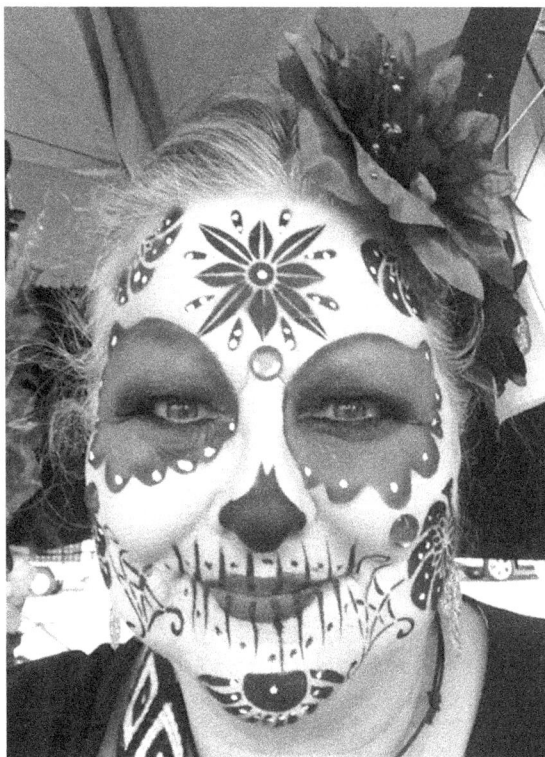

Author with Day of the Dead mask

Jungian Archetypes List

Carl Jung's theory of archetypes provides a framework for understanding universal patterns in human behavior and experience.

- **Hero** -The Hero archetype embodies the quest for identity and the courage to overcome obstacles. This archetype is often associated with the protagonist in myths and stories, representing the journey of self-discovery and personal growth. In everyday life, the Hero archetype can manifest as the drive to face challenges, set ambitious goals, and strive for self-improvement.
- **Mother** - The Mother archetype represents nurturing, protection, and fertility. It encompasses both positive aspects (care, comfort) and potentially negative ones (overprotection). This archetype plays a crucial role in our understanding of caregiving relationships and can influence our perceptions of authority figures and institutions that provide care or support.
- **Shadow** - The Shadow archetype represents the unconscious aspects of our personality that we tend to reject or deny. It often embodies traits we consider negative or undesirable. However, Jung believed integrating the Shadow was crucial for personal growth and psychological wholeness. Recognizing and working with our Shadow aspects can lead to

greater self-awareness and a more balanced personality.

- **Anima and animus** - The Anima (feminine aspect in males) and Animus (masculine aspect in females) represent the contrasexual elements of our psyche. Jung believed that integrating these aspects was essential for psychological balance and growth. Understanding these archetypes can provide insights into relationship dynamics, creativity, and the process of individuation.
- **Wise old man** - The Wise Old Man archetype represents wisdom, knowledge, and guidance. This archetype often appears as a mentor figure, offering insights and advice. In healthcare, patients may project this archetype onto experienced practitioners, seeking not just treatment but also wisdom and life advice. Practitioners can leverage this archetype to build trust and encourage patients to tap into their inner wisdom for healing.
- **Self** - The Self archetype represents the unified consciousness and wholeness of the individual. Jung considered this the central archetype around which all the others revolve. In healthcare, working towards integrating the Self can be seen as a journey towards holistic well-being, balancing physical, emotional, and spiritual aspects of health.

Feist, J., Feist, G. J., & Tomi-Ann Roberts. (2021). Theories of personality (10th ed.). Mcgraw-Hill Education

If inclined, you can find out about your archetypes by:

- *Asking, "What are my personal myths?"*
- *Identifying and listing your negative patterns. Be honest with yourself.*
- *Identifying and listing your positive patterns.*

Archetypes aren't good or bad, they're just patterns of behavior programmed into our subconscious. We have the power to change them.

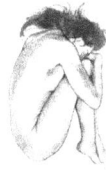

Chapter 8

Regrouping

Chakra #3 - Solar plexus - Personal power
and confidence - Color: yellow
Chakra #4 - Heart-love and compassion -
Color: green
Chakra #5 - Throat - Self-expression,
spiritual awakening, truth - Color: blue

The ending of my relationship with B meant that I was completely on my own without any financial support. While I welcomed this freedom, the responsibility of paying rent, feeding my dogs, and paying my bills wasn't something I had foreseen.

Penniless and without a work visa, I vowed to myself that I wouldn't give up living in Mexico. The house we had been renting had three large bedrooms upstairs, two smaller rooms downstairs, and three balconies, two in front of the house and the other in the back. The backyard balcony looked out onto a high wall that enclosed the large yard. The covered section of the yard was the perfect place for making handmade paper, which I had been doing for about four years.

I had to figure out how to make a living, fast! It occurred to me that I could rent rooms. I arranged the bedrooms and was able to find temporary renters, but I still needed more income to make ends meet. There was no other choice than to make artwork that I could go out and sell. Once again, I had to force myself to believe in myself, to stop fearing, and to stop thinking that I wasn't good enough.

Forcing myself to stop crying about my situation, I gathered the handmade cards I had been making in a nice basket. Praying someone would buy them, I walked into town. Walking from store to store, offering my cards. I met many people in town who asked about other things I made. My goal was simple: I needed to sell enough to buy food for my dogs. Success signified I would never miss paying the rent. Thankfully, I never missed a payment. Eventually, I added art lessons for both children and adults, photography, illustrations, painting, and handmade paper to my list of products. In addition, I exhibited in local galleries and art shows. Exhibitions led to a teaching position at a local university.

For the following two years, I remained focused on healing and making artwork as I reviewed my most recent past as if trying to remember a very complicated and bad dream.

During my teenage years and through my 30s, I had promised myself that I would never get married or have children. The examples I had seen growing up, witnessing my siblings and I living in a dysfunctional household, had been enough to maintain my resolve through my 30s. The reluctant human I had been born with couldn't justify bringing a child into a world of such chaos. In addition, my own desires to be free, travel, and experience life independently didn't seem like a proper environment to bring a child into the world. Accepting my own insecurities, it seemed unfair to bring a child into a world full of suffering and violence that I didn't understand.

Reconnecting

Having a fresh view of this wonderful and magical place that Mexico represented, allowed me to enjoy the new people I met. Soon, I made new friendships with other artists, expats, and locals.

I reconnected with a man I had met when I had first arrived in Mexico six years before (I will refer to him as T). T was married and had two daughters. Now, seeing him again and living in the same town, we met often for casual conversation. He had been separated for three years and was co-parenting his daughters with his ex-wife.

I was impressed with the loving relationship he had with his daughters, his kindness, and his soft-spoken demeanor. Although he had a traumatic childhood—abandoned by his mother at eight months old, never met his father, and had been emotionally abused by his adopted grandfather and spinster great aunts—what I saw was a man who had overcome his pain. T appeared to me as an exemplary father. About a year later, we found that we had fallen in love. We had our son soon after.

For the first time in my life, I felt hope for the future. I realized that I did have something to give a child; I had unconditional love. This child had come into my life to teach me love and so much more.

When I got pregnant, the youngest of my three brothers called my estranged mother and father, who had condemned and disowned me six years prior. He was the only sibling who had kept in contact with me. He shared the news with my parents. I believe his intention was noble; he told them that I had a husband and was expecting a baby. I wasn't entirely thrilled that my brother had contacted them. I left it up to them to do as they wished with the information.

My choice to follow B to Mexico had been a conscious choice that may have been less than ideal, but it had been **my** choice. I had struggled, but I had also enjoyed and loved life with B, particularly life in Mexico. Had it not been for B, I wouldn't have experienced the depth of the culture. Additionally, I lived happily without the condemnation of my parents.

Although I had forgiven my parents for the hatred and rejection they had for me in the past, I still had a fear of engaging with them. Therefore, I felt it was important to clarify my status. Before they assumed or jumped to conclusions, I wanted them to know that my relationship with a woman was just as respectable as it was with a man. I didn't want them to see my relationship with a man as proof of having been "healed" from lesbianism. Marrying a man and having his child didn't signify that I was "saved" from being a homosexual! It was an assertion that my ability to love wasn't about gender; it was about the person. I didn't want to be seen as the prodigal child who had returned in shame seeking atonement.

Some people may think it unnecessary to have confronted my parents with my personal ideological convictions. People may think it was too harsh, or that my parents wouldn't even understand. But I knew that if these issues weren't discussed, my parents would make assumptions that weren't true. When they banished me from their lives, I assured them that I loved them unconditionally. That's what I wanted from them now. Leaving myself open to getting hurt once again, wouldn't be an option. Avoiding the truth was **not** an act of love.

They could easily assume that I had finaly "repented from my sins" and that I had found the "right" path. The unconditional love they could bestow on me would be to acknowledge and accept who I was. Who I was wasn't a reflection on them. Gladly, we all respected each other and began to heal.

Completely unexpected and amazed, my mother surprised me with the wonderful gift of volunteering to come to Mexico for the preparation, birth, and welcoming of my son. She stayed with us for the traditional 40 days of quarantine to help me learn how to care for my newborn baby. I'll always be immensely grateful to her.

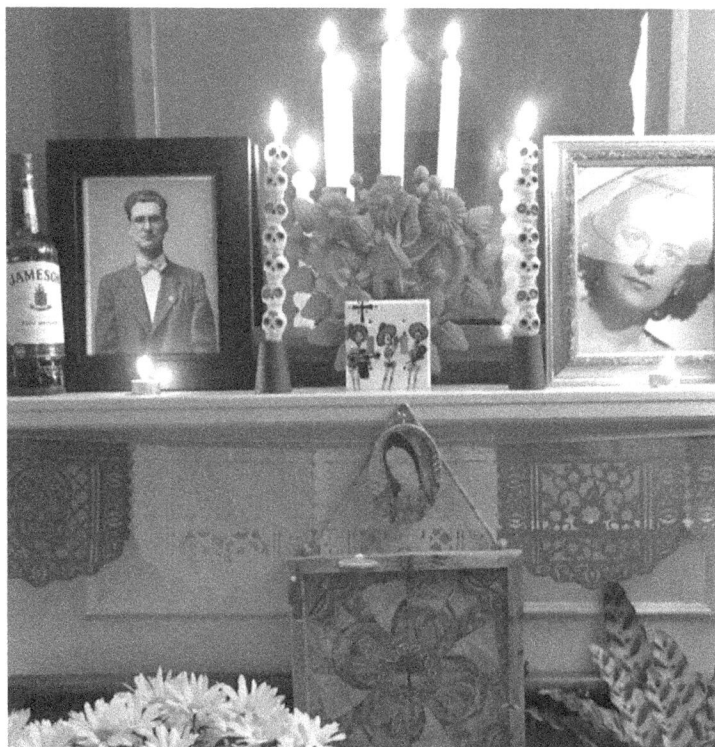

In honor of authors' parents, on Day of the Dead

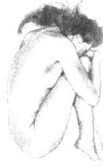

Chapter 9

Devaluation

Chakras - All

T had lost much of his capital with the arrangement he had made with his ex-wife when they divorced. As a result, he was forced to start a new business. My income from all of the things I made and my position at the university kept us afloat while T tried to build his small business. I had expected that his business would soon pick up, but by the time our son turned three, he was still unable to help provide for the household. To add to our problems, there was a significant devaluation in Mexico in 1995. This meant that my income alone was no longer enough to make ends meet. I panicked.

We decided that our only solution was to go to the U.S. We made a financial plan to go and work for five years. If we saved for five years, we would have more than enough to reinvest in our business and go back home. It required sacrifice on both our parts, but it would work. It was a very difficult decision for both of us; I didn't want to leave Mexico.

We agreed and I left first with my son. T followed a few weeks later.

We both found temporary jobs at first. Bilingual teachers were in high demand. Soon, I was hired as an emergency teacher. I was required to go back to school at night to fulfill the credential. The hours worked out well for me as it allowed me to pick my son up from school and spend time with him before I went to the university at night, when my husband could be with him.

Surprised that T had found a teacher's assistant position on his own, he later explained to me that he had been an elementary school teacher in Mexico City, something he had never shared. No wonder he was so good with children, I thought. Happy to see that we had adapted pretty well to our new routines, I felt confident that we would succeed in fulfilling our goals.

During the mid-1990s, there were so many students in L.A. that they created a system to rotate students throughout the entire calendar year. This way, they could accommodate all the students by creating a track system. T worked on one track while I worked on another.

Although I was exhausted, I was excited by my new career. Inspired by the opportunity to help the children of newly arriving immigrants, I looked forward to meeting them. Having just returned to the U.S. after eight years, I knew and understood these children. I had never imagined that both T and I would end up working with children, but I felt sure that with commitment, we could make a difference in these children's lives while working towards our goals.

The Body Speaks

When I was hired by the school district, I was required to get a physical evaluation. I was strong and athletic most of my life, but the evaluation showed that I had a malignant tumor on my thyroid.

Receiving this unexpected news alone stunned me. The word "cancer" was quite familiar to me since I had heard, spoken, and written "cancer" often for many years. Having worked in hospitals while I was in high school and university, it easily rolled off my tongue as if I were calling a longtime friend. But now hearing the word "cancer" referring to me, was incomprehensible. While my brain was trying to compute, all I could think about was my four-year-old son. I couldn't bear the thought of him growing up without me.

Hearing a very distant voice trying to explain something to me, the din of the doctor's voice slowly grew louder and clearer. "Thyroid cancer," she explained, "is one of the least deadly and most treatable of cancers."

Finally landing on her words, I heard the assurance in her voice. All would be well if we acted immediately. Surgery was scheduled for the following week.

After surgery, my doctor reported that although the tumor had begun to embed in my neck muscles, they were able to remove it with clear margins. After treatment and recovery, my doctor informed me that the tumor must have been there since I was at least 16 years old.

The thyroid diagnosis was a wake-up call. Since childhood, I felt disconnected from my body. I didn't yet understand the mind-body connection.

Someone who had heard of my hospitalization gifted me a book by Louise Hay, called "Heal Yourself Heal Your Life". This celebrated author from the 70s had healed herself and insisted that anyone could do the same. She also created a list of ailments and their "probable" metaphysical causes. It was a little too "woo woo" for me at the time. I found it interesting, but hard to believe.

Out of curiosity, I looked at **thyroid, possible metaphysical ailments.** *The following is what I found:*

- **Thyroid Gland:** *Humiliation.*
- **Throat Problems:** *The inability to speak up for one's self.*
- **Throat:** *Avenue of expression. Blocked channel of creativity.*

The issues associated with the **thyroid** *corresponded perfectly with emotions I experienced. It was curious that all the different alternative modalities of healing were related to emotions and thoughts.*

In my 40s, I was still afraid to express my ideas. The feeling of humiliation and fear to express anything was borne from the constant criticism that prevailed in my family. I can still hear echoes of the comments and humiliation remaining in my subconscious.

Louise Hay taught a seemingly easy and quick practice with the goal of developing self-love. You look at yourself in a mirror and say out loud, "I love you, I really, really, love you!" This was one of the most difficult things for me to do. It was so hard to get the words out of my mouth and then to say them. Each syllable was painful and awkward to utter. I felt stupid. The words didn't come out easily. In fact, it made me angry, and then it made me cry.

As I continued practicing daily, the tears finally turned into an attempt at a smile. My lips trembled and twisted into a weird and hilariously funny, awkward, grimace that made me laugh. Since then, I have embraced these moments with joy. It made me think of when I was a little girl and easily smiled. It's amazing that such a simple exercise can influence how you feel about yourself.

I had barely started teaching when the unexpected surgery occurred. I had to return to work as soon as possible, regardless of the lack of energy that prevailed while the hormones were re-adjusted. Thankfully, it only took a few months to feel renewed.

Our son had just turned five in early October, and although he wasn't too keen about Halloween, he was excited about Thanksgiving and, of course, super excited about Christmas. A few days after his birthday party, T informed me that he was going to Mexico for five weeks. His schedule allowed him a vacation in November and December. Understanding how much he might be missing his daughters, I encouraged him to go. But realizing that he had not considered sharing any part of the holidays with us upset me. I protested. He wouldn't change his plans; we would just make up the time when he returned. I let it go, thinking he must be very homesick and felt bad for him. I said nothing. We had agreed to speak every three days. He left.

My son would ask for his father daily. Then he began to cry incessantly, saying he missed his "Papi". Three weeks later, T called for the third time. He greeted our son first, then right after I took the phone, he told me he wouldn't be coming back. The youngest of his daughters "needed" him, and he couldn't return to the U.S.

At first, all my thoughts focused on helping his younger daughter, who I knew well. I offered to try and find a doctor in the U.S. who might be able to help, but he couldn't tell me what was wrong with her. Weeks passed with very disjointed conversations and less and less communication with our son. In the meantime, my son became more and more distraught while missing his father. The conversations kept going in circles as T continued to make excuses. *Maybe he was going back to his first wife,* I thought. No matter how many times I asked for an explanation, the answer was that he simply wouldn't return.

Finally, after a long three months, he confessed he simply didn't like the U.S. He wouldn't return. He wanted me to go back and join him. He had no job, no money, and no home. I had signed a contract with the school district, enrolled in evening classes to fulfill required credentials, and had bought a new car, all because we had made a commitment to our plan. Words cannot come close to expressing the shock I felt. I was completely shattered.

In the past, I had been able to see things coming, even foresee the end of a relationship. This time, I was utterly clueless, no warning, no nothing. How many times would I have to fall and get back up again? It felt as if someone had just told me that my husband had suddenly died. In fact, it was quite similar. They say time heals, but the wound I felt was painful and deep.

Truth Be Told

As time passed, I reflected as I carefully checked my emotions. Although I had immediately sought professional help to address how depressed I was, I still couldn't unravel my confusion. I didn't understand what had happened. Finally, through the lens of metaphysics, I realized that I had repeated a pattern I had seen my mother do.

When I was about 18, my mother confessed to me that after my parents' third year of marriage, she was very disappointed. She realized my father was not the ambitious or brave man she thought he was. She struggled with this fact.

One of the reasons my parents left Colombia was that my mother was worried my father would develop a drinking habit. As a sales executive, it was common in the day to negotiate deals over drinks. Moreover, my aunt worked closely with my father for the airlines, and they would often share a drink themselves.

My father and his sister had always been very close, but it was quickly becoming evident to my mother that her sister-in-law was overdrinking, although my father denied it. He would have a few drinks with his sister before going upstairs for dinner. By the time he came home, dinner was cold, and he had very little appetite. My mother was worried and aggravated that he, too, could become an alcoholic.

As a very young man, my father had the privilege of traveling outside of Colombia. He dreamed of living overseas, especially in the U.S., which he viewed as extraordinarily orderly and advanced, unlike the unsafe and chaotic city that was Bogota at the time. Seeking an escape, my mother craftily encouraged my father to seek an opportunity to improve her family's prospects.

I, too, felt disappointed in the man that I had chosen to have a family with. When I saw that T wasn't working enough to provide for our family, I thought of using my mother's tactic to give him a nudge and help him move forward.

I kept making excuses to give him a "chance" to adjust. For three years (the same amount of time as my mother had waited), I had supported him, hoping for change. Then Mexico suffered a strong devaluation, and I panicked. I had a three-year-old, and things didn't look good. I suggested we go to the U.S. just as my mother had. Reluctant to leave, I couldn't see any other way to survive the situation.

Thinking to myself, if he doesn't help financially once in the U.S., where it was easier to get work, then I had really made a big mistake. Would I have to leave him? But I couldn't really accept that possibility. I was married, the mother of his child, and I was committed to making this work. If I were a "good wife" and I truly loved T, I should be compassionate, patient, and accepting. I was a capable, modern woman, but I was still worried about asking for "too much", afraid to displease him.

Once in the U.S., T seemed happy, found work, and contributed to the household. We were starting to make money, and T was seemingly happier. I began to suspect that perhaps he was just unambitious like my father. Maybe I needed to accept him as he was. Rather than resenting T for his passivity, like my mother did my father, I needed to accept my husband as he was. The difference I neglected to acknowledge was that my father did, in fact, do everything he could, including sacrificing his dignity to support his family. T, on the other hand, wallowed in his misfortune and pride.

My son was deeply affected by the absence of his father. My greatest sorrow and concern was his well-being. Sadly, T had also repeated his own mother's pattern. He did to his son what had been done to him; he abandoned his son, just as he had been abandoned. Curiously, I felt stronger and more empowered alone.

You already know how this story ended. The important thing is that it ended. In fact, it was a blessing. I had repeated my mother's pattern subconsciously, encouraging T to leave Mexico in the hope of a better future. But my intention was never to stay in the U.S. Unlike my mother, I had the education, independence, and freedom to choose. Had I not had those qualities, I would have likely returned to the wifely duty of a struggling man. In addition, it was clear that in the United States, I could securely provide for my son. Recognizing that not all women had the freedom to leave their husbands, and deeply hurt, it was a "privilege" to deny his request.

Unprepared to be a single mother, the first thing I did was reach out for help. Thankfully, friends, parenting classes, and therapists for myself and my son were readily available.

I no longer trusted myself to make good choices when it came to choosing a partner. What had once been a hairline fissure in my heart from previous breakups deepened, forming a long, deep crack. The space in my heart that had once had a large capacity for love shut down. I was 41 years old and a love widow. Focusing on raising my son and becoming the best teacher I could be was my ultimate aim.

The story of my personal romantic relationships is clearly visualized in an illustration I once saw in a popular magazine. On the first page, there was a woman walking on a path. There's a hole on this path, and she falls into it because she wasn't looking. She manages to get out with some effort. She keeps walking. There's another hole, and once again, she misses it, falling right inside. She gets out again with a little less struggle. On the last page, there's yet a third hole, and guess what? Once again, she falls into it! This time, the hole isn't quite as deep. Nevertheless, she's in the hole, visibly exhausted, her hair messed up, and her bruised feet and elbows are resting on the edge while still in the hole.

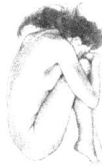

Chapter 10

Parenting

Chakra - Root - Security and stability - Color: red
Heart - Love and compassion - Color: green
Solar plexus - Personal power and confidence -
Color: yellow

My increasing stress and anxiety as a single and relatively older mother, simultaneously entering menopause, predisposed me to a possible crisis. I lacked the tools to face the challenge of a smart, impulsive, angry, young man. Unaware and unprepared to manage my son's complex behavior added to my existing stress.

The inability to communicate effectively with my teenage son affected me deeply. Desperate to find something other than talk therapy, which required years to resolve problems, I needed something I could do quickly.

A friend recommended I look into The Shift Network. The Shift Network provided courses in different areas of spiritual growth. Their goal is to empower and uplift people's lives. There, I found a class titled "Building Resilience" by The Institute of *HeartMath*®, founded in 1991 by Doc Childres.

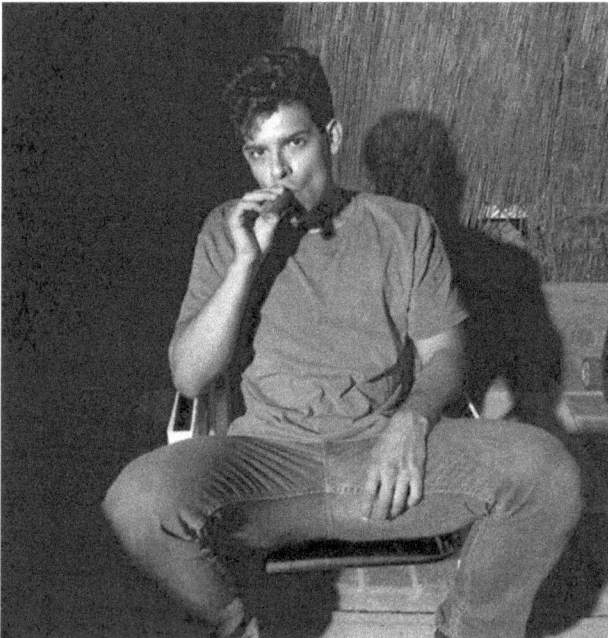

Author's Son

What is Coherence?

Our immune, hormonal, and nervous systems function in a state of energetic organization or harmony. The ideal state of the heart, mind, and emotions when synchronized and aligned is called "coherence". When we learn to activate renewing emotions like appreciation or kindness, then we can achieve coherence. When heart rhythms are in coherence, it helps the brain process information more efficiently. Thinking becomes clearer, and you can make better choices when you're in a coherent state.

As I practiced coherence, I could maintain my physical and emotional state without stress. Understanding the interaction of the heart and brain gave me the tools to increase my emotional resilience.

It's remarkable to experience that a simple breath before reacting to a stressful conversation with my son could make such a difference. Previously, I would react impulsively with anger, which would result in an escalated reaction from my son. Predictably, the result was a breakdown of communication. Using coherence even for a few minutes made a difference in the way I respond to stress in general. With the methods I learned in HartMath®, I gained tools to deal with my impulsive emotional reactions.

The methods employed in HeartMath® appear simple, but it's important to remember that learning something well takes practice and consistency. It's exciting to note that there are new developments in psychology and science that are being studied with quicker methods of success than traditional therapy. The Institute of HeartMath® is breaking ground in the area of technology as well, by creating apps and apparatuses to help us track our resilience. By measuring heart rate variability and coherence, we'll be able to bring awareness to what we once believed was uncontrollable without medication.

It wasn't until much later that I began to understand the complexity of my son's process of development. The development of boys' brains occurs much later than in girls. The pre-frontal cortex is located in the front part of the brain, and is responsible for developing the skills that require planning, prioritizing, and making good decisions. Sometimes this process may even delay maturity up to boys' late 20s or even 30s.

Thankfully, through consistent help for both my son and myself, we've finally learned to communicate in healthier ways. I'm happy to share that we're now kinder and closer to each other. While we were able to address our difficulties, there's an overwhelming increase in mental health issues in children from ages three to 17. Below is a chart that may help you identify and learn what may be going on with your children.

Facts from neuroscience	What does this mean?	Implications for practice
The frontal lobes are the last part of the brain to develop fully.	The frontal lobes govern reasoning, judgment, and impulse control, while other areas (including emotion centers) develop earlier.	Adolescents will act unreasonably at times, and explanations about decisions and consequences are unlikely to change their behavior. Young people will move between 'emotional logic' and 'rational logic'. This means we need to model and encourage thoughtfulness and problem-solving.
Dopamine levels shift during adolescence.	Dopamine links action to reward (pleasure). During adolescence, dopamine is moved around in the brain and is triggered by different things. Motivation lessens and things become boring, so new and risky behaviors are trialed to feel pleasure. Young people do things because they're dangerous. These risks are a normal part of developing a stronger sense of self, learning resilience, and developing mastery.	Risk in a developmental context is different from risk in a child protection context. Risk-taking behavior is an expected part of adolescent development. We can minimize risk by providing an underlying safety net and unconditional support. Our job is to facilitate good judgment wherever possible, rather than remove choices. We need to avoid ultimatums where young people lose face if they have shown poor judgment.

(Adapted from Jim Casey Youth Initiative, 2011, p. 20–24.)

Attention

For those young people who have been in care, the experience of transitioning to adulthood and navigating adolescence is further complicated by exposure to trauma and other early life adversities, including exposure to alcohol and other substances in utero, and neglect (McLean, 2016, p. 2).

If the core task of adolescence is to develop a strong sense of self, and the primary psychological effect of childhood trauma is to impair the sense of self, what does this mean for young people transitioning to adulthood? Puberty has been highlighted as an important time of neural plasticity. In contrast to the view that "the damage is done", experiences and interventions in adolescence can offset the effects of earlier adversity on the brain (Patton & Viner, 2007, cited in Robinson, Elly & Miller, 2012, p. 7).

Our role is to provide context, developmental experiences, safety, resources, and support for young people so they can move forward on their journey through adolescence to adulthood—at their own pace and in their own unique way. The process of planning is an opportunity to develop social and emotional wellbeing and positive outcomes for young people.

Reluctant Human's Thoughts on Parenting

I know that what I'm about to say is probably crazy, but after having to be a single mother and teacher for over 28 years, this is my idea for a possible solution to the problem of today's childhood crisis. I believe that the responsibility of having a child in our current North American society, with the emphasis on the nuclear family, the increasing number of single parents, and the new surge of children suffering from mental illness, means we need to create new rules. As I write this book, more and more children are experiencing mental health problems than ever before. I won't get into the many complicated reasons for this new phenomenon, but as a teacher and parent, I'm extremely concerned.

Aware of the controversy that I might instill, I propose a social system that requires prospective parents to learn how to parent, just like drivers have to have a driver's license to drive. The first license would be required for the prospective parents to take a course on the emotional needs of a child from pre-birth to four years old. They would have to renew every four years until the age of 18. I know this is a fantasy, but the lack of extended families nearby or trusted community members in a world that requires both parents or a single parent to work and leave the children without adequate guidance is creating a generation of emotionally ill-equipped adults.

Experience as a teacher has shown me the need in our modern society to address the diverse family structures that have evolved in the last 30 years. They simply don't meet the needs of our future citizens. This is a deeply concerning personal issue as a teacher and lover of our world.

A Need for Self-Reflection

*When I was younger, I used to think that when I met a new person I was interested in, I had to tell them my entire history. This way, I thought, they could begin to understand me, to know me. Becoming an adult, the stories were just getting too long to tell. Finally acquiring a little bit more wisdom, I realized that **I am not my story**. How liberating, because, in fact, I had been changing all along!*

We're not our stories. I don't mean to say that our stories aren't true or unimportant. I realized that we construct a narrative based on our experience. The story we tell about ourselves or others is a perspective of how we see the world around us. It's the perspective of us inside ourselves looking out. When we learn to become aware that there's a viewpoint coming from inside of us, that's when we find out who we really are. There's great value in stories and storytelling, but they're not who we truly are.

As a photographer, I often contemplated the question of how "true" the resulting image is. The moment you take the photograph, it no longer exists in real-time. It's an image stopped in time, never to be experienced again. In addition, many factors in a photograph can change the meaning, like the lighting, composition, point of view, size, and more. I find a similarity with the stories we tell ourselves. Maybe that's why we're so attracted to movies and visual media. Our brains have become, in a way, addicted to the "story". Some of us may struggle to contemplate, to enter that inner world, the world where knowledge, intuition, wisdom, and even guidance are waiting for us to listen or see.

Naturally, when we feel hurt by someone, our instinct is to react from our automatic fight-or-flight reptilian brain response. I've found that learning to ask my inner self questions before I lash out, surprised by an unexpected trigger, has helped me to avoid falling into a victim mentality. Asking myself these difficult questions, even if I was no longer involved with the person, helped me to see the hidden unconscious issue I had been perpetuating. What motivated my choice to get involved with this person? Did I choose to ignore a sign or clue? If I did something, why? Did I review my expectations before going forward?

I realized that I had chosen my partners impulsively, based on archetypes and patterns such as acting out the "mother" or "rescuer", which kept me in a constant state of anxiety. It was easy to keep falling into the "hole". Initially, I blamed myself for my lack of awareness. It took more work to finally understand and forgive myself.

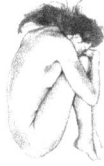

Chapter 11

Heart Break

Chakra #4 - Heart-love and compassion - Color: green
Chakra #5 - Throat- communication and truth -
Color: blue
Chakra #6 - Third eye intuition and insight -
Color: purple

The next 10 years proved to be particularly complicated and stressful.

At work, greater demands were being placed on teachers based on the political climate rather than the well-being of students. New mandates required teachers to focus on language arts and mathematics, prohibiting any other subjects from being taught, excluding science, social science, PE, and art. I felt that I was doing a disservice to my students instead of helping them. With this frustration and disillusionment, burnout would be inevitable.

When I first joined the school district, I had wanted to teach art in high school, but there weren't any positions available. I was encouraged to teach elementary school instead. After eleven years teaching elementary school, disillusioned with the new changes, rather than quitting, I searched for a position in other areas. Honored to be accepted in the arts education branch, I work with a wonderfully talented and highly professional group of teachers. I remained teaching art for another 10 years. Since it required that I simultaneously go back to school for another two years to get the credential, I decided instead to get a master's degree in art education, which required the same amount of time (two years) but gave me more options.

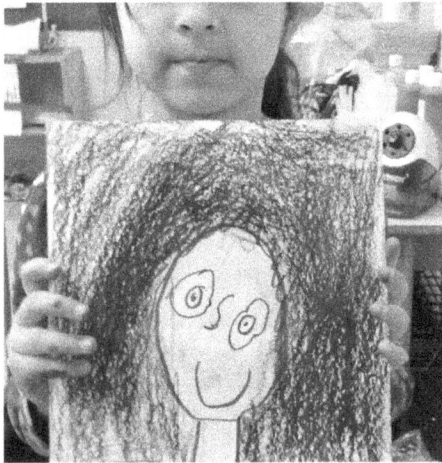

Student's self-portrait

Chac Mool

Chakra - Heart-love and compassion - Color: green

On my 50th birthday in 2006, I was determined to reconnect with the family my parents had left behind. It was time to heal the trauma of having been forced to leave my country of birth. My plan was to visit every year during my school breaks. Some of my aunts and uncles were still alive, and I had 35 cousins, a few I hadn't yet met. My desire was to reconnect and rebuild family relationships. I dreamed of moving back to live in a small village in the Colombian countryside. I had yearned to return so many years ago, but life had other plans for me.

During my first visit after 30 years, I was surprised to reconnect with a boyfriend I had when I was 17 years old. He was my cousin's best friend. I returned when I was 20, at which time he asked me to marry him. Still reluctant about the institution of marriage, especially in Colombia, since the customs were still very conservative and traditional, my answer was no. Now that we found each other again, 30 years later, both older, divorced, and a little lonely, our past history was rekindled. My heart was still fragile, but I thought I should give it a chance. Ignoring my intuition, once again I stepped into the "hole".

We formed a long-distance relationship for three difficult years. At first, we behaved like giddy teenagers in love again. During the school breaks, we took every opportunity to see each other. I hadn't been in a relationship for over six years. The long distance started to become too emotionally difficult. Realizing that we had both changed and that our priorities were incompatible, I began to pull away.

We hadn't formally broken up when suddenly I began to have shortness of breath and heavy bleeding, sometimes normal during menopause. Advised by health practitioners, I had a hysterectomy. Surprisingly, the tiredness and the shortness of breath remained.

At the insistence of a dear friend who had worked in the medical field and was married to a doctor, I went to see a cardiologist. I had just recently had a normal EKG, but my friend insisted I go see a good specialist. I obeyed.

The very thorough cardiologist examined me carefully and wasn't satisfied with what he heard. He ordered another, more invasive test. He found a very rare condition (especially in adults), so rare in fact, that it probably only occurred in one in a couple of million cases. I had a congenital growth underneath the ventricle of the aortic artery. It was obstructing 45% of my blood flow, clearly the cause of the shortness of breath. It was imperative that I have surgery as soon as possible.

But when I informed the cardiologist that my mother had been diagnosed with pancreatic cancer and was in hospice care, he immediately changed his mind. He decided it would be unwise for me to go into surgery at this time, due to the emotional stress I was under. He would wait until my mother passed. In the meantime, my directions were to keep as calm as possible, refrain from any lifting, and no unnecessary walking or exercise.

A couple of months later, my mother passed.

A Taste of Hell

The idea of having my heart cut open was terrifying. I focused on keeping my mind still, empty, and in the present moment. Yet, I couldn't remove the image of my chest wall being cut open to reveal my heart. Memories of my time in Mexico of the "Chac Mool", flooded my thoughts. *(The chac mool is an early Mesoamerican sculpture depicting an inclined figure. Individuals were sacrificed by having their blood and heart taken and placed on the offering on the stone figure.)*

Waking up in the recovery room to find my two lifelong friends sitting near me was comforting. The nurses began to remove the multiple tubes from my body. *Blue pill or red pill?* I wondered. I was Nemo from *The Matrix*, as they disconnected me.

Re-awakened with uncontrollable tears that wouldn't stop flowing, I realized my friends were no longer there. The anesthesia had completely worn off; the pain was unbearable. While I tried to get the nurse's attention, waving my hand because she wouldn't answer the call button, I tried to stand, hoping she would lift her gaze and see me through her window, but I was unsuccessful. Continuing to cry in agony, she completely ignored me. Then, finally, she looked up, still on her gold mobile cell phone, and yelled at me from her glass-caged perch as she continued chatting, "Stop crying!" she yelled, "You should be grateful you're alive!"

Trying not to cry because it made the unbearable pain in my chest even worse; I felt completely alone. Hooked up to IVs, nauseous, unable to speak from the pain in my chest and heart, insulted in addition to being yelled at by a soulless witch, was a special kind of hell.

When finally leaving the hospital, I was given a nice, stuffed, red heart-shaped pillow, signed by my surgeon and his assistant. It was a considerate gesture since the purpose of this pillow was to hold it against the chest, in case of coughing or sneezing. Whether or not I had just been through one of the most barbaric experiences in my life or one of the most amazing examples of modern medicine, I felt like I had been run over by a train or two.

Once home, I slowly hobbled to the entrance of the front door and glanced at the large, ornately carved wooden Mexican mirror that stood next to the living room wall. There stood a pale, small, hunched-over, approximately 99-year-old ghost of a woman. She was looking at herself, as if she had just returned from the grave. It took a second or two to realize it was me looking at myself.

Purgatory

I remained highly emotional during the first week post-op. Despite taking the medication, the pain wasn't diminishing. A good friend drove me to the post-op appointment just one week later. As she was driving, we hit a relatively small bump in the road. I screamed in pain as I felt a deep stab in my chest. We were close to our destination. Seeing that I was entering the office bent over, moaning, the doctor realized what had happened. He sent me to get an emergency x-ray as he called ahead to warn my surgeon and the hospital.

The sternotomy, which was secured to the chest wall with wire sutures, had somehow come apart. A bacterial infection acquired in the surgery room had made my bones soften enough to loosen the wires. I couldn't believe this was happening! What had I done to deserve this? Back to surgery. Undo, debride, redo! Double whammy!

Donning my newly acquired ensemble, which featured a handy IV clutch bag, antibiotic kit, easy-on/off oxygen tank, and a lightweight accessory spirometry tube, I arrived home from the hospital in full regalia. It was too painful to cry, and I was too shocked to talk to anyone, so I remained silent, quietly trying to regain a little sense of humor. Complete physical recovery took about a year, but the trauma still haunts me sometimes.

Almost every human being has had their share of trauma of varying degrees at some point in their lives. I wasn't aware of this fact until recently. I thought that "trauma" was reserved for war veterans, severe physical tragedies, or accidents.

It wasn't until I experienced the heart surgery that I learned about post-traumatic stress syndrome. After the procedure, I couldn't control my unending sorrow. The daily crying, which in my mind was unwarranted and inexplicable, was exhausting.

One day, I met a man who came to my door to set up a neighborhood program for our area. When I opened the door, I suddenly broke out in tears. He kindly asked me what was wrong. I apologized and explained that my recent emotional state was uncontrollable due to my heart surgery. He proceeded to share his own story of post-surgery trauma after having heart surgery. Helping me understand, he validated my experience as traumatic. Full of gratitude, I thanked this unexpected visitor angel that had appeared and comforted me when I was feeling most alone.

Meditation and spiritual practice helped me regain my emotional strength. Surprisingly, during this process of healing, I discovered other emotional blocks that I had never imagined were "traumas".

Today, there's a lot of information and treatment that address many forms of trauma. Sometimes, just becoming aware of the origin of the trauma is healing in itself. In addition, it is important to remember that trauma resides in our bodies, affecting our brain, heart, and gut.

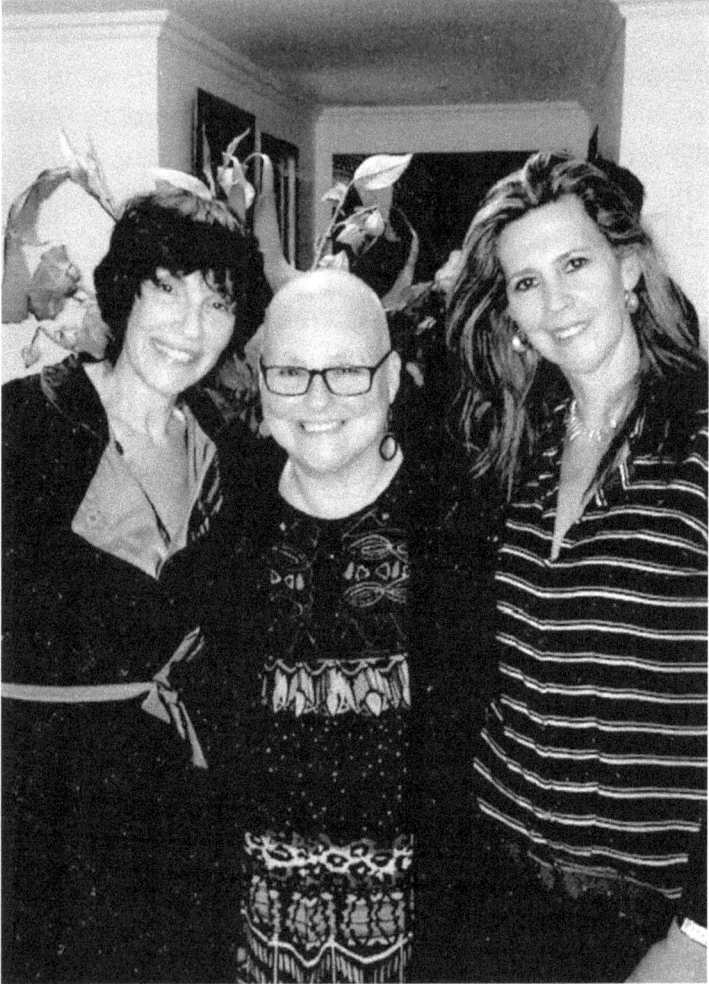

Family

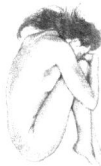

Chapter 12

Overwhelmed and Done

Chakra #4 - Heart-love and compassion - Color: green
Chakra #5 - Throat-communication and truth -
Color: blue

The end of 2016 was a busy and memorable year. It was the year I turned 60, two years short of retirement, my son graduated from university, and Donald Trump was elected president.

Teaching became more and more challenging as the implementation of technology was mandated in the classrooms. Many teachers began to leave the profession due to the stress put upon them. Both the politics in education and constantly changing mandates resulted in growing teacher dissatisfaction and disillusionment, a fact that affected me deeply.

For the last two years, I had been working overtime, accumulating 10 to 11 hours of work per day, including prep time and transportation time. After my regular assignment as an itinerant art teacher with the school district, I visited students in their homes who were in a Hospital Home School Program. I committed to this schedule in order to pay for my son's university room and board. This allowed him to graduate without any debt.

My son entered university, which offered me a respite from both our reactive behaviors. But when he returned after graduating, we fell back into conflict. Raising a boy by myself gave me the opportunity to resolve my difficulty in understanding men. Unfortunately, they still remained an enigma.

Reproaching myself for the inability to stop the emotional drama and thorny communication, I became depressed, lonely, and helpless. I blamed myself for the mistakes I made, and I blamed my son for his lack of sensitivity and understanding. Traditional therapy wasn't helping. I simply gave up, exhausted; it was easier if I just died.

Driving home from work one winter day, I received a call from my doctor's office. I had just had my yearly breast checkup the previous week. It was my doctor's nurse. I pulled over to answer the call; my heart was pounding, forewarning my fears. She proceeded to give me the results of the test. She said that I had a rare breast cancer and I needed to come to the office as soon as possible.

"It can't be!" I exclaimed.

I asked her to please confirm what she had just said. Once again, she repeated and added, "The test result on the report says that you have metaplastic breast cancer, stage 4."

I was told to call immediately and make an appointment to see the oncologist. I was stunned, but not surprised. Sitting parked in my car, feeling overwhelmed with all the stress I was experiencing both at work and at home, I cried quietly for a few minutes, more from exhaustion than sorrow. What I felt was relief.

Experience has taught me the importance of taking someone with me when going to the first appointment for a major medical issue. Someone who can offer emotional support is great, but ideally, it should be someone who can also take notes, think of questions to ask, and most importantly, record key facts the doctor is saying. When diagnosed with something as serious as cancer or any other life-threatening illness, always take someone. I was usually alone at my doctor's visits. I could have saved myself a tremendous amount of grief, fear, and loneliness—had I reached out for help and allowed myself to be vulnerable.

The next day, a dear friend accompanied me to my appointment. Prepared with a list of questions and acting as my patient advocate, she made me feel cared for.

As the young doctor began the consultation, it was clear that he hadn't expected to have to answer so many questions. My friend was not only married to a respected and well-known doctor but had also worked in the medical field most of her life. The objective wasn't to intimidate him; it was to ask the right questions in order to maintain clarity and establish good communication. Since my previous experiences with surgery hadn't been ideal, having someone to help me was crucial.

The conversation with the oncologist wasn't smooth. He was put off by most of our questions, perhaps because he was intimidated, or maybe he was just concerned that he had passed his allotted 15 minutes of patient time.

I'm forever in deep gratitude for both my lifetime friend and her husband. They took the initiative to investigate and find a possible clinical trial for this rare metaplastic breast cancer. Their timely research found the only two existing clinical trials in the U.S. One was on the East Coast, and the other one in San Diego, California. These amazing and generous friends not only went out of their way to source the information but also booked an appointment for me to see the doctor in San Diego! The visit to the specialist and researcher in San Diego

*told me there was a possibility that there could be one
last hope in case the chemo failed.*

The last few years had been so emotionally exhausting
that it was easy to accept the possibility of the sweet
slumber of death. Although I wasn't suicidal, I was
extremely emotionally exhausted from the pressures
of life unfolding before me. Life was simply too hard.
Even though I was unable to cope, no tears were shed.
Looking forward to resting in peace, ready to surrender,
I wasn't afraid of death. This truth didn't cause me
sorrow; on the contrary, I welcomed it.

There was no cure for rare metaplastic breast cancer,
but my prognosis offered a three-year life expectancy
if I accepted the chemotherapy treatment. Upon
calculating the possibility of living up to the estimated
three years, I imagined it would give me at least a
little time to be free to make art. Even if the chemo
was simultaneously killing me, I could still create. The
thought of this prospect emboldened me.

My inner "reluctant human" had been nudging me to do
nothing, take the chance, reject the dreaded chemo,
and leave my body alone as I had previously planned.
On the other hand, I no longer had the obligation to
work. Consequently, I could dedicate whatever spare
energy I had to my passion.

The "standard of care" for metaplastic breast cancer
triple-negative stage 4 requires removal of breast
tissue, then chemotherapy. The nurses called this

type of chemo "The Red Devil" because it was one of the most toxic. At first, I tolerated it. By the second-to-last session, almost six months later, I could no longer endure the poison.

Upon ending the chemotherapy treatment, I remembered that when I lived in Mexico, many years ago, I had met a few expats who had survived terminal cancers after visiting the Hippocrates Institute. Later, they moved to Mexico to live a less stressful life, thriving in remission for many long years.

I was still weak after ending chemo. Regardless, I used a portion of my retirement savings to go to the Hippocrates Institute in Florida. Following their example, I attended the recommended three weeks in this beautiful place. I didn't expect to be healed. My goal was to eliminate the horrible toxins from my body.

I spent my time enjoying the beautiful and serene gardens, wheat grass treatments, colonics, nutrition classes, bedside hot sauna, ice water and hot pools, massage, wellness seminars, ozone treatments, and much more. Three weeks later, I felt well enough to embark on my mission to Colombia.

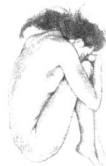

Chapter 13

Going Home

Chakra #6 - Third eye intuition and insight -
Color: purple
Chakra #7 - Crown-spiritual and universal
consciousness - Color: gold

It had been my wish to retire and live in Colombia. Now I wanted to end my days in a small town or village in my country of birth. With the help of my youngest brother, his adorable daughter, and my close friend, we embarked on our mission to find a home. I knew that my days were numbered, but I was serene as I visualized myself thriving in the peaceful surroundings of my prospective new home.

Three days later, my eyes started to bother me. Uncomfortable because I hadn't brought my sunglasses,

I just closed my eyes when it got too bright. It was the tropics after all. We found a beautiful house that we all liked and put in an offer. My eyes seemed to be getting worse by the day. I only got headaches when it was time to get new glasses, which is what I suspected.

My brother, his daughter, and my friend all had to return to the U.S. That morning, I woke up with the same headache. By the time we were on the road back to Bogota, the pain in my head had gotten worse. Driving in the beautiful green and changing countryside during our four-hour drive, I looked forward to the serenity of trees and wildlife my new yet shortened life would provide. I closed my eyes and tried to continue dreaming.

Approximately two hours into our trip, little blue dots of light flashed in and out of my right eye as the pain increased. Upon arriving in Bogota, my brother and friend went directly to the airport and departed. I had planned to stay with a close cousin to wait and hear from the realtor's office. I could no longer tolerate the pain in my head. Fortunately, there are several doctors in my family. My cousin immediately called one of them. When he heard my symptoms, he ordered her to take me to the emergency department immediately. By this point, the pain was unbearable, and the little cerulean blue dots increased, flashing before my eyes ferociously.

Doctors first suspected an ocular migraine. To confirm, they did a CT scan. When the test result arrived, it revealed a brain tumor. A rock falling on my head would have been softer than this news. I had been looking forward to the possibility of living three more years, and now I felt my impending death.

As my heart sank, so did my legs and body. Reaching back onto the gurney, I grabbed onto the rails, holding on as I sobbed. The shock was great, and the sorrow was deep. Tears, fear, and frustration previously absent in the last diagnosis released themselves, gushing onto my face, violently choking as I cried.

Then, I heard in my right ear a soft and gentle voice say, "But you said you wanted to die. We were just doing what you wanted, trying to make it faster for you." These words were loud in my ear and deep in my heart. No longer crying, in that instant, I knew that whatever happened from that moment on, I truly had to change. I had to appreciate every moment, find love in everything, let go of disappointments, let go of my arrogance and cynicism, release the "reluctant human" and embrace whatever moments I had left. Seeing how ungrateful I had been, I asked for forgiveness from myself and the divine creator of all things, for the lack of appreciation I had for the beauty in life.

The doctors in Colombia were very concerned and honest. They assured me that the best thing to do was to return to the U.S. immediately. Colombia's doctors are excellent clinicians and surgeons, but they lack the sophisticated, state-of-the-art equipment to treat complex brain issues.

Deeply saddened and afraid, in less than 24 hours, I boarded my flight from Bogota to Los Angeles. Thankfully, my cousin's husband, a physician, had supplied me with ample steroids to keep the swelling down in my brain, the cause of the headaches. From the airport in Los Angeles, I was immediately taken to the hospital. The surgeon suspected metastasis in the brain due to the breast cancer, a common occurrence. He believed that since the brain tumor was in the visual area, there would be a chance of losing my eyesight.

Living in Gratitude, No Matter What

The thought of losing my vision was frightening, especially since I was an artist. In an attempt to minimize my fear, I thought about my years in art school. I had imagined what it would be like to lose my vision. In one of the art classes, we were given an exercise that taught us how to see things with our mind's eye. We were asked to practice drawing several ways without looking at the subject, sometimes by touch, others by drawing from memory, feeling textures without seeing them, etc. Surprisingly, our eyes aren't the only way to see. I had imagined I could use my sense of touch to sculpt. The memory of that mental image offered me some solace, just in case.

After recovering from surgery, I was wheeled back to my room, still under the influence of steroids and remaining anesthesia. I lifted my arms with elation. I announced to everyone as I entered the ward, "I can see! I can see! I CAN SEE!" In fact, I was truly very happy that I could see. Those who knew me smiled since I was normally quiet. Everyone laughed and applauded, sharing my joy.

The updated diagnosis was a new primary tumor, not what the surgeon had first guessed. It was not metastasis from the breast cancer. What the doctor found was a tumor located in the left occipital lobe of the brain, the area of the brain in charge of the visual field. My probable lifespan was now reduced to 18 months. The standard of care for glioblastoma multiforme wild type is a very light, easy oral chemo for six weeks and targeted laser radiation to the area of the tumor. Both were a breeze compared to the breast cancer treatment.

Sleep had never been a problem for me, but what I began to observe was that as the suture wounds healed, I remained extremely tired and lethargic. I was unable to stay awake for more than one hour. I slept four hours for every one hour of being awake. Constant sleepiness can be just as tormenting as not being able to sleep.

My inability to stay awake was unbearable. What kind of life was that? After expressing my frustration to my oncologist, he put me on Adderall, a stimulant that helped me stay awake. I didn't like having to take pills, but it allowed me a better quality of life. Living with two terminal illnesses required a very different way of living.

Having promised myself that I would become more aware of all the beautiful things life had to offer, I needed to change the way I thought. The switch happened almost instantaneously. As soon as I heard the message, I focused on the present moment. I couldn't afford to live any other way. When I woke up in the morning, the first feeling was surprise, and the next thought was gratitude.

Knowing that my first goal was to maintain being present in mind, body, and spirit, I could sense a connection (although I didn't understand it) with spirit. Spirit spoke to me and woke me up.

Still battling with my thoughts, looking to make sense of things, and more so with a body I didn't connect with, indicated I still had many things to resolve. Since the tumor was in the area of the occipital lobe of the brain, it affected my right visual field. This meant that when I looked at something through my left eye, I could see fine. When I looked through my right eye, the image flicked on/off, and back and forth, making it impossible for me to drive or read. Eventually, I got used to it, but it's still annoying.

I used to have difficulty adjusting (and still do) to the fast-growing advances in technology that have emerged in my lifetime. Often, I've complained about the loss of the "simple days". But when it comes to modern technology that allows people with disabilities to be able to have access to knowledge and joy, I'm deeply grateful.

Most of the books that I wanted to read were available in an audio version. The alternative to reading visually has given me the opportunity to continue studying and "read" faster. Multitasking had never been as enjoyable as I often "read" while cleaning or doing other simple tasks.

Having resolved both the sleeping and the reading problems, I was prepared to continue my research and art.

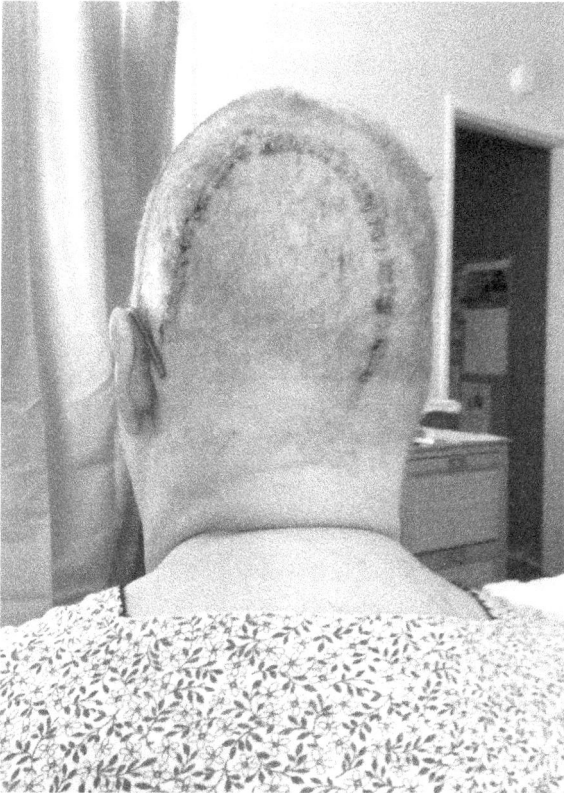

Brain scar

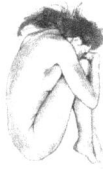

Chapter 14

Planning for the Inevitable

*Chakra #6 - Third eye intuition and insight -
Color: purple
Chakra #7 - Crown-spiritual and universal
consciousness - Color: gold*

Right after returning home from the hospital, my first task was to put my affairs in order. My youngest brother came to help me with all of the legal documents I needed to put in place in the event of my death. This was very important to me because I had heard horror stories of families that were unprepared. Lack of communication regarding our personal issues often results in unexpected conflict. Having everything done and clarified makes it easier for the remaining family members.

My parents followed the tenets of Catholicism. They taught us that we had a soul that was eternal and that our body was temporary. We never cease to exist. As a reluctant human teenager, I just couldn't accept what I didn't see. When I got older and started working in a hospital, I experienced several patients in the process of dying. That experience proved to be profound.

It was evident to me that when someone died, something actually left the body. Einstein's theory of energy, $E=mc^2$ (where energy equals mass times the speed of light squared—the scientific explanation that proves that energy cannot be destroyed or created, it can only be transformed) clearly proved to me that if we're made of mass and energy, when we die, what appears to be left is the mass/flesh, but the energy that's released from the body remains. It cannot be destroyed.

If we're made of energy (invisible) and mass (visible), the energy has to come from somewhere. I believe that's the essence of what we are, energy.

Both my parents are gone. My mother became extremely stressed as my father's cognitive condition declined. She was in denial of his Alzheimer's diagnosis. Although she was his main caregiver, she refused to get help. As my father's disease progressed, my mother's ability to cope diminished. She was convinced my father was behaving like a child to aggravate her. I could see her frustration and anger building as my father's cognitive abilities faded. I'm certain that the stress she endured was more than she could handle. The anger and resentment my mother acquired evolved into a diagnosis of pancreatic cancer. She died within one year at 79 years old in 2009.

My relationship with my mother was complicated and difficult. Although we had mended our relationship when she had come to help me during the birth of my son, she still did and said hurtful things. I had stopped reacting when in her presence, but her toxic behavior hadn't changed. When I returned to the U.S., I could only be around her for a very limited amount of time. I loved my mother, but it would only take about 15 minutes to get triggered.

My mother died without ever saying she loved me. As an adult, I understood that it was common for my generation to have parents similar to mine, but my inner child didn't understand this. In addition, I had never been the daughter she wanted me to be. I wasn't good enough in her eyes.

On the day of her funeral, my role was to stand outside the church to guide people to an alternate entrance because the main church was under construction. After everyone entered the church, I stayed outside pretending that there might be some stragglers. My mother had been brave, generous, and liked by many, but I had been too emotionally battered to forgive her. My anger was too deep to have to endure listening to her adulations.

After my mother's death, my middle brother took the responsibility and most of the burden of my father's care without complaint. I tried to help when I could. My father had lived with Alzheimer's and dementia since the age of 70. When it became impossible to care for him at home, we were forced to take him to a convalescent home. He was there for only two months of his life. He died peacefully in his sleep at 89 in 2011.

The difficulty of witnessing my parents' deaths wasn't the most problematic. Instead, it was the frustration of witnessing the insensitivity towards patients in our medical system that was sometimes cruel and sad.

My three siblings and I faced our parents' process of dying alone. We had never experienced death in our home. As adult children of immigrant parents, it was challenging to manage both the necessary paperwork and their care. For me, the witnessing of their death was a natural process. They had prepared us to see it as such. I'm grateful for that because, regardless of the sadness and loss felt, I believed as they did, there was something beyong death. They had the conviction of their religious belief. I relied on science, what I had seen in the hospital, and what my gut said. There most certainly was something more after death.

Immediately after the brain cancer surgery and treatment, I discovered Dr. Joe Dispenza's website and ordered his first meditation. The meditations I had learned in yoga classes were short, lasting only five to 15 minutes. Dr. Joe's meditations lasted much longer, from 30 minutes to over an hour! Now in 2017, he was offering classes online and creating live events. Since I was unable to read due to the loss of my right visual field, I resorted to listening to recorded books, which was a blessing. I took all of the courses that were offered online because they were affordable. Unfortunately, I was unable to afford the in-person seminars, but I diligently studied and meditated an average of three times a day.

Six Years Free

Contrary to expectations, I survived six years passed both diagnoses. I outlived the diagnosis of metaplastic breast cancer past five years, at which point my breast oncologist said I was considered in full remission. The glioblastoma multiforme didn't reappear for an extremely rare six years. Throughout most of those years, I had MRI exams every two months, then every three months. I made a significant amount of artwork during that time, used up all my savings traveling, and continued studying all things regarding healing and metaphysics while expecting sudden death at any moment.

In my quest to understand why my body suddenly decided to manifest so many different strange illnesses in the second half of my life, I approached my investigations as an unsolved mystery. While seeking motivation, I also wanted to find a solution. My inquisitive mind kept me equally engaged in learning about subjects that intrigued me, like the modalities of healing both in cutting-edge modern scientific areas, as well as in the areas of spirituality and mystical traditions. Studying has by no means made me an expert, but it has opened a world of possibilities I knew existed and are worth exploring.

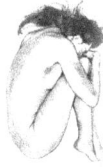

Chapter 15

Peaceful Surrender

Chakra #5 - Throat communication and truth - Color: blue
Chakra #6 - Third eye intuition and insight - Color: blue
Chakra #7 - Crown spirituality and universal consciousness - Color: gold

In order to improve our living situation, we needed to do some remodeling. My son was prepared to take responsibility for managing the work. Excited about the project, I didn't foresee all that it implied. I neglected to consider the inconvenience that occurs when doing construction while living in the home. The noise and interruptions alone were enough to cause me anxiety. Consequently, my stress increased, and I began to feel sick.

Despite having survived longer than expected, I still had lingering physical issues. Unfortunately, chemotherapy and other treatments leave debilitating conditions that may never return to normal. Therefore, I still have to watch my energy levels. The unexpected jarring sounds, rhythmic pounding noise, interruptions, and general construction problems proved to be too much for me. I could sense my energy draining. The impact on my energy and stress levels were reflected in the next MRI, the tumor had reappeared.

Having witnessed my parents' death, assured me that I didn't want to die in a convalescent home. Nor did I want to be a financial burden on my son or my three busy brothers. I was immeasurably grateful for having been given these extra and unexpected six years of life. My first thought was to enroll in the end-of-life program available through my health plan.

My neuro-oncologist insisted on one last attempt at chemo. I rejected his offer. My veins were practically destroyed, but he insisted that oral chemo should be easier. Against my intuition, I tried it. My body rejected it violently. It only took three days for me to realize that I could no longer tolerate any more treatment. I never wanted to be touched or poked again. To which my neuro-oncologist replied, "Oh, that's ok, it really doesn't work anyway!" His response not only made me feel angry, but also like I was his lab rat. I entered hospice immediately after rejecting any further treatment.

My hospice doctor was wonderful! One of the most caring human beings I've met. I felt calm, waiting for the will of the Universe patiently, for my last earthly moment to arrive, as I held on with love in my heart.

Since I had been admitted to hospice, my neuro-oncologist had calculated that I would have to take the medications to end my life. That date was to be set on September 28, 2022.

By August, I had declined very quickly. First, I started to get shaky and lose balance. Soon, I needed a walker, and then, I was reduced to a wheelchair. Problems with speech were next, first forgetting words, then words that simply refused to come out correctly, which made for some pretty funny mistakes.

Eventually, I gave up talking on the phone because I just couldn't get words out quickly enough for a conversation. It was exactly as my beloved hospice doctor had explained when I had asked him what the death process would look like in my case. He said it would be like an Alzheimer's patient. In the end, the Adderall would no longer work; I would just sleep a lot. Fortunately, the brain doesn't feel pain unless it's swollen or if a patient is put in an awkward position during surgery.

For the last six years, I had loyally followed Joe Dispenza's teachings and meditations three times a day. Unable to afford his seminars, I dreamed of attending one day. In the meantime, I continued to follow him on social media.

One day, while in hospice, I checked online and found a post from Joe Dispenza calling for patients for one of his trials. I immediately applied and was accepted!

This particular trial was for "Remote Coherence Healing". The trial consisted of receiving remote healings from his vetted group of healers once a week for three months. Stool sample and spit sample kits were sent to patients to collect and submit each month. On the healing days, I was instructed to connect to a live recording of a special meditation online. The meditation included vibrational electronic sounds embedded in the music for approximately one hour. The healers were given a photograph of me and a diagnosis that they could use while they were connected to the call. I never saw them, nor did they see me. Just the electromagnetic energy that connected us was sufficient.

Enormously grateful to have found this opportunity, I didn't assume I would be healed. I knew that things aren't always in our hands. I surrendered gently to this truth, yet I was open to the possibility that there are things that exist that we cannot understand or see.

The Coherence Remote Healing began the first week of August. There was no evidence of change the entire month. I had no set expectations, so I wasn't discouraged. I focused on the meditation, which was soothing.

In the second month, I began to have movement in my arms and legs. My head started to bob side to side and shake uncontrollably back and forth. At first, I was frightened, but then I remembered the videos of the testimonials that I had seen online. I relaxed and let my body do its thing.

Very slowly, I began to feel a little bit better every day. By mid-September, the nurses were reporting that they were confused because they saw I was minutely better every day. Incremental changes continued to reveal themselves daily. I was getting better. By the second week of September, I no longer needed help to bathe.

September 28, 2022, was the big day! The day to review the result of the last MRI and be ready to plan the ingestion of the medications to end my life with dignity. The doctor and the neuro-oncologist I had known and seen for the last six years, every three months, was expecting to confirm the advanced growth of the tumor. The size of the tumor would indicate the appropriate time to administer the end-of-life medication. It was critical that I be aware to take the medication while conscious and able to swallow.

We were used to meeting online and viewing the results simultaneously. One time, we were both surprised and scared while we were looking at a scan, but he had pulled the wrong patient by accident; the name didn't match. Now, as we looked simultaneously to review the MRI scan, he was speechless. I could see that he was confused and was rechecking his information. I suspected this might happen, but I remained quiet. He still said nothing, as he fumbled around looking at his computer.

Finally, I asked, "What's wrong?"

He said, "Nothing."

Another long pause, then he said dubiously, "The tumor has decreased," he finally answered somberly.

Since he continued to just look at the scan, I asked, "Is this normal? Does this happen?"

He answered back curly, still looking at the scan, "No, absolutely not!"

He was visibly astounded and speechless. (*This is a research doctor, mind you.*)

I asked next, "What should I do?"

Finally lifting his head to look at me, he said, "OK, call and make an appointment in six months."

Unbelievable!

A combination of shock and happiness ran through my body and mind. Shocked because I couldn't believe the lack of concern or even polite interest in what could have reversed the growth of the tumor. The doctor I had joked with, made an art piece in his honor, and shared information about brain cancer, had nothing to ask me, nothing positive to say. I was saddened and disappointed, and frankly, I was angry. I never heard from him again. I never went back to his office, nor have I had an MRI of my brain since.

As of today, I'm still healing and thriving. Some residual damage due to the initial surgery still affects my right visual field, making me unable to drive. Otherwise, my walking ability has increased, and I no longer need a cane. The newfound energy and continual recovery are astounding. Each morning, I wake up with immense gratitude, and each evening I go to sleep grateful for another day of life. I continue to recover and feel better every day. Minor issues like the need for medication for neuropathy, naps, Adderall, and difficulty with vision still persist.

The Visitation

One day, several years after both my parents had passed, I was in a deep meditation when suddenly, I felt the need to open my eyes and turn my head to my right. Both my mother and father appeared in a sort of transparent bubble and surrounded by a vignette of light. Only their shoulders and heads were visible. My mother greeted me gently and lovingly. Unexpected tears quickly ran softly down my face.

I asked my mother how they were, and she answered, "Very well and happy!"

My father was farther away and I couldn't see him clearly. When I asked how he was, he zoomed in closer, covering my mother's face. He also said he was, "Very well and very happy."

I wanted to "hear" more words, but was too overwhelmed to ask. They looked younger and healthier. Although I heard nothing else, they spoke to me telepathically. We apologized to each other for the pain we had all caused each other. There was so much more I wanted to say and ask. But instead, we said our goodbyes. Gentle tears continued to run down my face; they disappeared. Neither of them had ever said they loved me, but for the first time, I believed I had just heard them say it. I felt their love deep inside my heart.

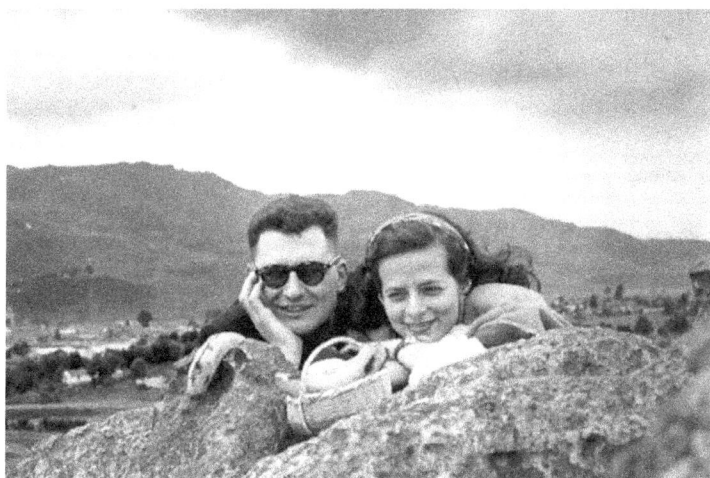

Author's parents

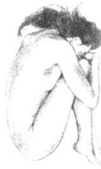

Chapter 16

About Life

I'm aware that I've made many mistakes as a partner and mother. I'm also aware that it takes courage to face our demons. The irony is that those demons are created by our own negative thoughts and speech.

Without having had the clarity to understand my life, my experience of reality was a series of bombarding sensations of all kinds. Growing up in the city with unending noise, traffic, sirens, honks, construction, loud music and sounds, people, machines, airplanes, trains, etc., was overwhelming if not dehumanizing.

As an art student, I enjoyed exploring and photographing the "concrete jungle" of the warehouse districts and commercial buildings away from the city or suburbs. Yet, the farther from nature I was, the more reluctant I was to appreciate life itself. I valued authenticity, but what I saw in most people in my city was a lack of originality and a building desire for more and more superficial things. These were the thoughts that occupied my mind as a young and developing reluctant human.

When I initially read or heard that the purpose of life is to learn, I didn't quite get it. First, I thought, well, duh! Of course, we have to learn, but is that really all that life was about? My mistake was that I was focusing on intellectual learning, like going to school and getting a job, so that we could survive. Then, I realized that the experience of life was built into the experience of learning. Everything that's alive has to learn. All living creatures follow this truth. Our senses—vision, touch, taste, sound, and smell—are the tools with which we primarily learn. Then life experiences teach us the more nuanced and complicated lessons. To add to the mix, we have emotions, and emotions like our senses are all made of energy.

It seems ironic that when we're born, we're entrusted to learn everything from our parents and the existing social paradigms. In the process of experience and maturation, we struggle with the incongruities of the things we've been taught. Then, in the process of becoming more aware, we realize that we have to unlearn the patterns we were taught. Perhaps that's the whole purpose of looking for truth. Truth changes as we change. We inherit the unresolved problems in order to facilitate evolution. If one generation doesn't succeed in resolving the problem, perhaps the next one will. We live on the surface of the *experience of life for most of our lives. Any added stress blocks our energy, which eventually gets depleted. These are the moments when we respond impulsively to negative emotions and thoughts. We often make judgments or assumptions that aren't entirely true.*

Perhaps a culture that practices a metaphysical path is a way to learn to become "better" humans. How amazing would it be if we could learn to build consciousness as soon as our brains are able to learn?

About Thoughts

As I mentioned in the beginning, as a child, I believed everything was possible. I couldn't believe the world was as fixed as everyone said. Somehow, somewhere, everything existed or could be created. Slowly, as time passed, this idea faded as I was mocked due to my lack of logic.

I don't know how much of my original belief may have influenced the reality I now live in, but once again, a greater part of me believes that we live in a world of infinite possibilities.

Our thoughts are "heard" by our own brain. Our brain acts upon what you tell it and think. Yes, it hears your words and follows your thoughts. Therefore, it's very important to be careful with your thoughts or words. Just like a child, your brain will take everything you say or think at face value. Thoughts come from our subconscious mind, which occupies the smallest portion of our brain.

The unconscious part of our brain is where the largest amount of data is stored, holding all of the past memories and information. Buddhist monks know this. That's why in their practice, they talk about "right thoughts and right speech" (in addition to other principles). The aim in all mystical practices is to achieve consciousness.

About Resilience

I was raised Roman Catholic, but as soon as I saw the incongruity of different teachers' interpretations of the lessons, in addition to witnessing the hypocrisy and behavior of both clergy and parishioners, I rebelled. I left the church, not the mystical teachings. Although I abandoned the church, and frankly most of the connection to it, I maintained interest and curiosity for the essence of the mysticism of the spirit. It sparks questions in me to the degree that I enjoy learning about other mystical beliefs. Throughout my journey, I have been guided more and more to the mystical, to the degree that I'm not afraid of death. I surrendered to it, peacefully accepting the unknown.

When life seems difficult, I try to imagine a positive outcome. I know, it's not easy, but just pretend at first. With time and practice, you can change your thoughts and your life. I'm a living example of this. Remember, your brain is listening, so you need to keep reminding it of who's in charge. Our minds are more powerful than we have been led to believe.

Don't be afraid.

Don't give up.

Perhaps the answers that we're looking for as human beings will be found as we move closer through the lens of the mystical or spiritual. Science is slowly melding with previously lost ancient knowledge, holding the promise of a better future. Just like the "miracle" of my survival, our world can also heal. We just need to surrender fear, build resilience, open our hearts, and seek to live authentically.

Dear and beloved humans, may we all go bravely forward.

Self-portrait on bucket list trip

Recommended Reading

Dr. Joe Dispenza: *Evolve Your Brain, Breaking the Habit if Being Yourself*

Dr. Bruce Lipton: *The Honeymoon Effect, The Wisdom of Cells*

Dr. Mario Martinez: *The Mind Body Code*

Dr. Gabor Maté: M.D., Psychologist: *The Myth of Normal, Hold On To Your Kids, The Retrn to Ourselves*

Paul J. Mills: *Science, Being and Becoming*

Phillip Moffet: *Dancing With Life*

Anita Moorjani: *Dying To Be Me*

Dr. Sue Morter: *The Energy Codes*

Carolyn Myss: *Medical Intuitive and Teacher: several, Arquetypes, Anatomy of the Spirit, Why People Don't Heal*

Oliver Niño: *Spiritual Activator: Do This Before Bed*

Dr. Judith Orloff: *Empath, The Genieous of Empahy*

Suzanne Scurlock: *Body Mind Connection, Healing from the Core*

Alternative Healing Modalities and Treatments I Tried:

Acupuncture

Ancestral work

Chakra Balancing

Energy Work

Epsom salt baths

Gerson diet

Hippocrates Institute

Hypnosis

IV Glutathione

IV Ozone

Reiki

Trauma Work

Additional Information

During my lifetime, I've witnessed more advances and changes than my parents did in theirs. I implore everyone to take responsibility for their own health, mental and physical. Our health system is broken, no doubt about it. It behooves us to learn more about our bodies, especially since we're experiencing concerning issues in our health system.

Fortunately, we're entering an era where science and the metaphysical are beginning to blend. Some pioneers in this are people like Deepak Chopra, Dr. Sue Morter, Dr. Joe Dispenza, Dr. Beth Dupree, and Dr. Bruce Lipton. I'm sure I have missed others.

There are many teachers emerging right now, coming out of seclusion after being ridiculed, judged, or shamed. Some are still considered too "woo woo". Others have been practicing for a long time and secretly work with famous celebrities, actors, billionaires, politicians, and even heads of state.

If you're looking for a slightly different approach to healing, a good starting point may be to look for a functional medicine or integrated medicine practitioner. Homeopathy is excellent for children and adults. Holistic medicine, osteopathy, hypnotherapy, and acupuncture are others you can try.

Last but not least, there are both practitioners and modalities that can be healing. There are people who teach you how to heal yourself. Some healers offer everything from energy work, breath work, meditation, herbs, paranormal healing, shamanism, psychic healing, medical intuition, and much more. For a list of more resources please visit my website: www.adrianamunozhernandez.com

About the Author

Adriana Muñoz Hernandez was born in Bogota, Colombia, in 1956. Her parents emigrated to Southern California when she was six. She was raised and educated in Los Angeles. She received a degree in fine art and in biology.

During her early years, she worked in hospitals and began exhibiting photography in galleries. Moving to Mexico at 30, she continued her art, exhibiting, and teaching both privately and at the Universidad Valle de Mexico.

Upon returning to California, she became an elementary school teacher for 11 years. Finally, she returned to her art via teaching as an art education specialist for another 11 years.

Adriana Muñoz Hernandez has always had an insatiable curiosity about the human condition. Leaving her country of birth was a traumatic experience for the highly sensitive six-year-old. As a result, she developed into what she called, *A Reluctant Human*.

In 2017, she was diagnosed with a rare, terminal metaplastic breast cancer. Eight months later, she was diagnosed with a separate cancer of the brain, glioblastoma multiforme wild type. Currently, she lives in both Los Angeles and in her native country, Colombia.

In Gratitude

In everlasting gratitude to my son—thank you for your patience and help when my brain would go "offline". To the illustrators, my dear lifelong friends, Anne London and Dusty Atkins, who whip up masterpieces at the flip of a brush. To an amazing duo, Natasha and Stuart, and the entire crew at *The Ultimate 48 Hour Author,* thank you for your patience, encouragement, and professionalism; you made my dream come true. To my incredible teacher friends, who have been there for me unconditionally in my most difficult moments.

I love you all!

Notes

_____

_____

_____

_____

_____

_____

_____

_____

_____

_____

_____

_____

www.ingramcontent.com/pod-product-compliance
Lightning Source LLC
Chambersburg PA
CBHW022058020426
42335CB00012B/741